The Manual That Should Have Come With Your Body

*You Only Have One Body
and It Must Last
a Lifetime*

CINDY HEROUX RD

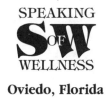
SPEAKING
SOF**W**
WELLNESS

Oviedo, Florida

Library of Congress Cataloging-in-Publication Data

©2003 Cindy Heroux RD
ISBN 0-9745609-0-1 (trade paper)

Publisher: Speaking of Wellness
2200 Winter Springs Blvd. Suite 106-202
Oviedo, FL 32765

Cover photo by Beverly Brosius
Cover design by Andrea Perrine Brower
Inside design by Dawn Von Strolley Grove
Production Management by Sandy Dolan

This book is dedicated to my parents
Beryl and Angelo (Lou) Maggi
who by example, both good and bad,
taught me the value of living a healthful life,
and to my husband
Marc
and my daughters
Katie and Kristin
for their love and support.

CONTENTS

Part One: Basic Operating Instructions

I. EAT

II. MOVE

III. RELAX

IV. SLEEP

Part Two: Important Safety Precautions

Part Three: Preventative Maintenance

PREFACE

Why You *Need* This Manual for Your Body

When you buy a new car, computer or even a washing machine, you are provided a manual, a set of instructions that gives you clear, concise, and important information that will help you to keep your new product running well and assure that it will last as long as possible. Thanks to a manual you know what type of fuel your car needs, how much pressure should be in your tires, and when you should take your vehicle in for routine service and preventative maintenance.

Your body is more complex than any machine you could ever purchase, but it didn't come with a manual. It didn't come with a warranty either. This is unfortunate because you only have one body and it must last a lifetime. If it breaks down or ages prematurely, you don't get to trade it in for a new one, and replacement parts are very hard to come by.

Since you are going to live for the rest of your life, taking the best possible care of this one and only body that you have is of paramount importance. The choices you make about what to eat, how much exercise and rest to get, and whether or not to smoke or take dietary supplements, will determine the quality of your life both now and in the future. But what is the best way to care for your body? What kind of fuel will help your body's engine to run most efficiently? What type and how much exercise do you really need to maintain health and ward off disease? Is not getting enough sleep a minor inconvenience or a cause for serious concern? There is so much information out there, much of it conflicting, that figuring out exactly what you need to do to keep you're your body running smoothly and operating at peak performance can be difficult. I have written this Manual to make it simple for you. The Manual That Should Have Come With Your Body contains the basic instructions on everything you need to do to live a healthy, happy, and productive life presented in a down to earth manner and a simple to use format.

Based on the latest research combined with common sense, The Manual explains what, when, and how much you need to eat, move, relax, and sleep. It also explains what *not* to do and why. It doesn't pretend that there are any easy or miraculous answers to achieving better health, or to losing weight, because there aren't any. Most fads and magic pills are temporary fixes at best. At worst, they can be dangerous or distract you from doing the things for your body that will make a real difference in how good you feel, how great you look, and how long you live. The Manual isn't a weight loss book because you don't need one. If you make lifestyle choices that encourage overall health and wellness, your body weight will adjust on its own naturally, unless you have a medical condition that prevents it from doing so. It also isn't a medical book or intended to replace getting advice from your health care provider, especially if you do have an existing medical condition. Rather it is intended to be a starting point towards living a healthful life and preventing illness and injury.

If you follow the Basic Operating Instructions in this Manual, heed its safety precautions, and see your health care professionals for routine service and maintenance, you will be doing everything you need to in order to be healthy and achieve wellness.

"Wellness . . . the state of physical, mental and spiritual health that allows you to live your life to the fullest and realize your greatest potential"

Cindy Heroux

ACKNOWLEDGMENTS

I would like to thank everyone whose love and support helped this book to become a reality including my family, friends, and neighbors who took time to listen to me, read my work, and provide valuable feedback. I would especially like to thank Shelley La Marre for suggesting such a wonderful title, and Bill Pickering for providing the motivation and opportunity to bring this book to print.

INTRODUCTION

YOUR LIFE IS IN YOUR HANDS

Good health gives you the freedom to enjoy your life to the fullest and to seize every opportunity that comes your way. When you are well, you have the energy and ability to follow your dreams, and to participate and take pleasure in everything around you. You feel great, look wonderful and are strong enough to face the challenges of life. Good health is truly one of the greatest gifts you can possess. If you doubt this at all, talk to someone who has lost their health, or think back to how miserable you felt the last time you had the flu. It was probably very difficult for you to participate in life or enjoy much of anything at all. When you are sick or in pain nothing else seems as important as feeling better and getting well again.

Many people underestimate the value of their health until it begins to fail. They avoid making healthy choices a priority until a medical crisis arrives like a wake up call. Even then they may look to medicine for a magic pill or a miracle cure rather than to their own lifestyle for answers. Yet it is your lifestyle and the day to day care of your body that has the most power to affect the quality of your life, both when you are feeling fine and when illness or injury strikes. The success of magic pills and miracle cures is still dependent upon the underlying health of the person who receives them.

Health and wellness don't just happen, they must be encouraged, maintained, and protected, and the only person who has the power to do that is you. It is up to you to take the necessary actions to create optimum health and reduce your risk of illness. Just ask your doctor! As we come to better understand the significance of lifestyle in health and disease, even the focus of medical care is shifting towards the importance of prevention.

Early in the twentieth century, most people died from infectious diseases such as pneumonia and smallpox, or from industrial accidents. Thanks to the development of antibiotics, vaccines, and other "miracle drugs," together with advances in surgical procedures and technology, we have effective treatments for many of these ailments today, and survival rates have improved. While infections and injuries are still an important concern, the greatest threats we now face are from chronic illnesses that develop over time, such as heart disease, cancer and stroke. Rather than being caused by something outside of ourselves, the development of these chronic illnesses is primarily related to our family history and the lifestyle choices we make each day. We can't alter the genes we inherited from our parents, but whether we choose to eat right or not, to remain active and exercise, or get enough rest, can strongly influence the expression of those genes. The *way* we choose to live our lives can determine how long we will live, and what the quality of our lives will be.

Preventing illness and injury is far less painful, less expensive and more convenient than coping with illness or injury, and the disruptions they can cause in your life. As the old adage says—

an ounce of prevention is worth a pound of cure—in today's world, it may be worth much more.

There are separate but overlapping roads to creating health and preventing illness and injury: lifestyle management and early medical intervention. The lifestyle management road involves making healthy choices like those outlined in this manual. They help you to build a strong, healthy body, and limit your risks of developing disease. A healthy lifestyle can help you to avoid many health problems altogether and delay the onset, or minimize the severity of others. When a health issues does arise, early medical intervention can slow its progression, help to prevent it from becoming an even bigger issue, and reduce the chance that it will negatively affect other aspects of your health. Both lifestyle and early intervention are important, but the more time and energy you invest in a wellness oriented lifestyle, the less medical intervention you are likely to need.

Because lifestyle management and making healthy choices requires more time and effort to improve your health, it is often the road less traveled. Some people would rather take a dozen drugs a day than have to change the way they eat or make time for exercise and rest, but there are distinct advantages to a wellness lifestyle over medical intervention. There are no serious side effects to be concerned about, it is less expensive, more rewarding, and more powerful; it improves your total health rather than one aspect of it. There are effective drugs that can help lower your cholesterol, ease your heartburn, and help you to fall sleep, but none of them has the broad, global power to make you feel your best, look your best and improve the overall quality of your life that living healthfully does, and they *do* have serious side effects that you should be concerned about.

Consider the difference in your options for treating an

elevated cholesterol level. If your cholesterol level is too high, it increases your risk of developing heart disease and having a stroke. To lower your cholesterol, you could eat a healthy diet that is low in saturated fat, high in fiber, and includes lots of fruits and vegetables. You could move more, sit less, exercise regularly, and learn to manage stress effectively—or you could see your health care provider and start taking a statin drug such as Zocor or Lipitor.

If you choose the lifestyle changes and stick with them, your cholesterol level will probably drop significantly *and* your ratio of good cholesterol to bad cholesterol will improve. But the benefits won't stop with your cholesterol and your heart. You will also reduce your risk of developing cancer, diabetes, and obesity. Eating right and remaining active will improve how well your brain works, your kidneys function, and your bowels move. A wellness lifestyle can help prevent blindness, improve the texture and appearance of your hair, skin and nails, and lead to a better sex life—and those are just the highlights. That's a pretty impressive return for investing some time and energy in living well!

On the other hand, you could just take a statin drug which would lower your cholesterol, but you would miss out on all of the other benefits that come along with a healthy lifestyle. There is one thing though that statin drugs do offer that lifestyle changes don't—side effects. While your cholesterol numbers may fall, so may you, due to muscle weakness and pain, known as myopathy, a known side effect of statin drugs, which in some cases can progress to muscle breakdown, kidney failure and death. Other possible side effects include neuropathies, or nerve related problems, and cognitive issues such as memory loss. There really is no such thing as a free lunch.

I'm not saying that you shouldn't take statin drugs and that they don't have their place, but even the National Institutes of Health National Cholesterol Education Program guidelines recommend initiating lifestyle therapies *first* and only adding drug therapy if the goals for improving cholesterol aren't met through these lifestyle strategies. Unfortunately, most health care providers receive far more training in the use of drugs than in the areas of wellness. More importantly, most have more confidence in the likelihood of their patients complying with their recommendations of taking medication than in their patients making permanent lifestyle changes. The constraints of today's medical system also don't allow most health care professionals the time to talk about lifestyle changes or supply patients with the information and support they need to make them. The easier solution is to write you a prescription and send you on your way. It's convenient for everyone, but may not be the best choice when it comes to your overall health, especially if it discourages you from taking steps towards living a healthier life.

Medical interventions such as statin drugs have prevented thousands of heart attacks and saved many lives, especially of those people who are at high risk for heart disease, but they should be used *in addition* to a healthy lifestyle not in place of one. Swallowing pills may be the road that most people take, and it may seem easier than changing the way you live, but in the beautiful words of Robert Frost . . .

Two roads diverged in a wood and I—
I took the one less traveled by,
And that has made all the difference.

Choosing a wellness lifestyle can make "all the difference" for you too! If you invest time and energy in a healthy lifestyle, it will greatly improve your chances of aging gracefully with vitality and good health. Making healthy choices for your body doesn't guarantee that you won't get sick, but it definitely improves your odds of maintaining health. Taking the time to see your health care professionals for regular exams and health screenings is also important. They can provide guidance in deciding what the best choices for you are and offer early medical interventions that are appropriate when necessary.

A HOLISTIC APPROACH

Working towards wellness is a holistic approach to health that capitalizes on the interconnectedness and interdependence of your body's parts and systems. If you are having chest pain, feeling depressed and fighting a cold, you might see a cardiologist for the chest pain, a psychiatrist for the depression, and a family doctor to treat your cold and flu symptoms, and each would likely prescribe a treatment plan appropriate to one of your conditions. The cardiologist might prescribe a drug or recommend further testing. The psychiatrist might offer anti-depressant medication and therapy, and your family doctor would probably tell you to rest, drink plenty of fluids, and possibly take an antibiotic.

However, if you are experiencing problems with your heart, your emotions, and your immune system is weak, there is quite likely an underlying health issue such as poor nutrition or excessive stress which is contributing to all three. While you need the medical care to deal with the immediate symptoms, making the lifestyle changes that would address the underlying issue could help to improve all three conditions at once, and help you to feel better overall.

A wellness lifestyle also takes into consideration the inter-connectedness of your mind and spirit with your physical health. I once had a physician tell me that the back pain I was experiencing was "All in my head," as if my head were somehow disconnected from what was going on in the rest of my body. It was his sincere belief that if there was an emotional or psycho-logical issue contributing to a condition, it somehow made the symptoms less real or less relevant. Gratefully, medical profes-sionals today are more enlightened and recognize that the effects of stress can have a profound effect on your physical health. It is well documented that stress doesn't just make you feel tense, nervous or emotionally drained; it changes every-thing about the way your body functions, from blood pressure to brain chemistry, and is a very real cause of physical illness. A wellness oriented lifestyle takes things like stress and inter-personal relationships into consideration. It addresses the needs of your mind, your body and your spirit by building on the fundamental principle that whatever is happening in one organ or system in your body affects every other organ and sys-tem in your body, and your health in general—positively or negatively.

I've explained how broad and powerful the impact of healthy choices can be, but it's helpful to remember that the reverse is also true. When you abuse or neglect a part of yourself, the rest of you will suffer as well. Consider smoking. We most often asso-ciate smoking with lung cancer and emphysema; a direct cause and effect relationship—you put bad stuff into your lungs and bad things happen to your lungs—but the damage doesn't stop there. Smoking also contributes to atherosclerosis in coronary arteries reducing the blood flow to the heart, damages blood vessels, and makes the blood stickier, dramatically increasing your risk of having a heart attack. It reduces the amount of oxygen available to your muscles making strenuous activity and exercise difficult, and it breaks down the collagen in your skin causing increased wrinkling. Knowing what *not* to do is just as important to your health and wellbeing as know what *to* do.

Since all the systems in your body work in harmony with each other and contribute to your total health, your choices can also have a domino effect. Eating well will provide the fuel necessary to get the most from your workout. The harder you can work out, the more stress it will relieve and the better you will sleep. The better you sleep, the more energy you have to do the things you want to do (including more exercise), and to cope with the challenges of life. Better nutrition and more exercise also lead to better weight management. Better weight control reduces your risk of diabetes and heart disease, and can give you a more positive feeling about yourself. Feeling better about yourself can improve your outlook on life as a whole and a positive attitude will improve your relationships and your work. One good thing leads to another.

That's why the instructions in this manual are so valuable. Every single step you take towards caring for your body moves you a little closer to looking great, feeling your best, and achieving optimal health.

The younger you start taking good care of your body, the better, but wellness works at any age. If you begin in your twenties or thirties, it will help you to preserve the strength and vigor of your youth. If you are middle aged, it can keep you fit and healthy and feeling great. Even in your eighties you are still capable of building more muscle, strengthening your heart and improving your flexibility.

USING THIS MANUAL

The best way to use this manual is to read it cover to cover because each section contains a great deal of valuable information and builds on the section which precedes it. It also follows a logical order of progression. You must first have the raw materials with which to build a healthy body; these come from your diet. Many of those materials will be used to build and maintain a strong body through movement. Then you must make sure that stress, or a lack of sleep, don't undo all of your hard work. Finally, you must protect your health and your body from harm. That means both paying attention to the safety guidelines and performing routine maintenance checks. Once you are familiar with the information, you can use the individual chapters as reference guides and the "KEYS" as check lists to see how well you are incorporating healthy choices into your life.

I am sure that you will already know some of what you find on the following pages, but I am equally certain that there is information there that will be new to you, because thanks to ongoing research, our understanding of health is constantly changing. So turn to the Basic Operating Instructions and get started at living well and taking the best care of your body possible!

PART ONE:
BASIC OPERATING INSTRUCTIONS

I. EAT

1

YOU REALLY *ARE* WHAT YOU EAT

E very cell, tissue, organ and system in your body is built out of the foods you eat. Food provides the building blocks that you are made of, the replacement parts for maintenance and repairs, and the fuel to keep you running. If you provide your body with the right foods, in the right amounts, at the right times, your body will reward you with better health and smoother operation. People who eat well also feel well, look well, and have more energy with which to enjoy life. They are more resistant to illness, recover faster from injury, and they are better prepared to handle all of life's challenges.

A healthy diet doesn't just affect your body, it also affects your mind. Good nutrition can help prevent depression, reduce the symptoms of Attention Deficit Disorder, and slow the progression of Alzheimer's disease. It can soothe your soul when you are upset and provide the power to help you compete. It may even make the difference between aging well and getting old before your time.

With each bite that you take, you are determining the health of your body in the present *and* in the future. Making sure you get enough calcium will help to keep your heart running smoothly today and your bones strong tomorrow. The reverse is also true. Consuming lots of soft drinks high in sugar may cause you to gain weight today and the phosphoric acid they contain may contribute to your developing the frail bones of osteoporosis when you are older. Nutrition is a powerful ally in the creation of optimum health and the prevention of disease when you use it to your advantage.

Eating healthfully isn't difficult to do. It simply requires giving your body what it needs and avoiding the things that it does not. First and foremost, your body needs enough water and fluids. Without sufficient fluids in your system, the importance of everything else becomes secondary. If you do nothing else this manual recommends other than make sure you drink enough water every day, you will be taking a giant step towards better health. Secondly, your body needs fuel for energy, and the raw materials with which to build and repair itself, including carbohydrates, proteins, fats, vitamins and minerals. Each of these nutrients is equally important in keeping you healthy; without enough, or with too much of any of them, your health will be compromised. Your body must also be protected from substances which can cause damage, like trans fatty acids, excessive amounts of alcohol, and harmful chemicals. Following the guidelines in this section will help you to accomplish all of this.

WHEN TO EAT

You were born with a wonderfully efficient internal mechanism designed to make sure that your body gets what it needs, when it needs it. As a baby, you ate every three to four hours, not because you had a tiny stomach—your stomach was just the right size for the rest of you—but because your body was *designed* to eat every three to four hours. You were responding to a signal from your internal mechanism that said you were hungry and needed food; a signal that you were still very attuned to.

Unfortunately, as they get older many people stop listening to their bodies and learn to respond to external signals instead. They train themselves to ignore or override their internal signals in order to make life more convenient, to accommodate the expectations of others, and to please their senses. Instead of eating when they are hungry, many people eat because "it's time to eat," even if it happens to be several hours before or after they really need to. They eat because someone else says they should, or because something looks or smells so good that they "just have to." People even eat just to give themselves something to do when they are bored. These are *not* good reasons to eat. While you should certainly enjoy eating (I love food so much I majored in it in college!), the only reason to eat is because your body needs refueling. You don't overfill your gas tank or expect your car to run on empty and you shouldn't expect your body to either. Healthy eating means tuning back in and learning to listen to the wisdom of your body rather than what the outside world has to say.

When you tune back in, you will likely find that your body feels best and operates most efficiently when it is fed smaller amounts of food spread throughout the day rather than two or three large meals. Starting out your day with a healthy breakfast and having a light snack before you go to bed are helpful too. Breakfast literally means break-fast, the ending of a period of not eating. When you wake up in the morning, your body has gone several hours without refueling and is in need of nutrients. A healthy breakfast jumpstarts your metabolism and provides the fuel your body needs to function well throughout the morning. Because your body does much of its maintenance and repair work while you are sleeping—this is also when children grow—a snack before bed helps to ensure that your body will have enough raw materials to work with.

Frequent meals eaten when they are needed helps stabilize your blood sugar levels and can make it easier to resist overeating or succumbing to temptation. One reason why coffee bars and cookie shops are placed near the entrances to food courts is because you can smell them from a great distance. Their enticing aromas make your mouth water and your stomach growl, tempting you to come hither and eat. It's a great marketing strategy that counts on the power of suggestion being able to trigger your appetite even if you aren't hungry. Maintaining a constant blood sugar level will make resisting temptations like this much easier. It will also help you not to eat too fast. Have you ever arrived at a restaurant feeling like you were starving and devoured an entire basket of chips or rolls that were sitting on the table before you even ordered your meal? Waiting too long between meals can encourage this kind of explosive eating and increases the chances that you will eat more than you need.

How Much to Eat

How much you eat is just as important as when or what you eat. If you eat more than what your body needs, even of the healthiest foods, you will gain weight. Obesity is a full blown epidemic in this country. It affects children as well as adults and is a major factor in most of the chronic illnesses you are hoping to avoid. Obesity is a complex problem with many contributing factors, but right at the top of the list along with lack of exercise, is portion control—or should I say, the lack of it. The notion that more is better simply doesn't apply to good nutrition.

Enough is better than more!

Portions sizes have gotten out of control, especially in the foodservice industry. Because customers sometimes equate quantity with value, restaurants often serve oversized portions to make their patrons feel like they are getting a "good deal." But when you order a meal at a restaurant and they serve you a portion that's large enough to feed a family of four, it really *isn't* a good deal unless you share it with three other people or take it home and use the leftovers for three more meals. You may be getting more food for your money, but you are paying for those large portions with your life—literally. Oversized portions make it difficult to control how much you eat, and overeating leads to weight gain. Weight gain can lead to diabetes, sleep apnea, heart disease, and may increase your risk of cancer.

Over time you may also be paying for large portions out of your wallet. American's spend billions of dollars each year on weight loss products and services, and even more money dealing with the health consequences of obesity. When you consider the big picture, including the economics related to your health, large portions aren't necessarily the bargain they appear to be. When you eat out, try ordering smaller portions, like a lunch size for dinner or an appetizer as your meal. If you do order a whole meal, share it with a friend or put the extra food that you don't need to eat in a "to go" container before you begin to eat. That way you won't be tempted to eat more than you want or need.

PERSONALIZING YOUR PORTIONS

Recommending standardized portions would be fine if people came in standard sizes but they don't. What might be an appropriate serving size for a petite woman who weighs 110 pounds and spends most of her day sitting at a desk might only be a snack for her 220 pound brother who plays football. Nor do people carry around scales and measuring utensils in their pockets. The best and simplest way to determine the right size portion for you is to let your own body be your guide.

Meat, Poultry and Fish: Choose a serving about the size and thickness of the palm of your hand. Removing the skin or visible fat will help you cut back on calories.

Beans and Legumes: As a main dish, a good serving is about twice the size of your fist. For a side dish, one fist should be enough.

Dark Green and Brightly Colored Vegetables: As long as you are leaving room for the other foods you need, it's hard to eat too many vegetables, so have all you care to as long they aren't cooked in fat or covered with sauce. Even though cauliflower isn't brightly colored, it belongs in this category.

Starchy Vegetables: Vegetables like potatoes and cassava should be considered more of a starch than a vegetable and should be eaten in smaller quantities, no more than the size of your fist.

Fruit: Fruits are healthy, but can be high in sugar. For dense fruits like apples and pears, one fist is fine. For watery fruits like watermelon, use two fists.

Grains: If your grains are a side dish, one fist is plenty; if they are the main dish, you need two, and whole grains are always the better choice.

Nuts and Seeds: Nuts and seeds are high in fiber and very healthful, but they are also high in fat so only eat as much as you can hold in the palm of one hand.

Fats and Oils: Partially hydrogenated fats should be avoided as much as possible, and saturated fats like butter limited to the size of your thumb from the middle knuckle forward. Unsaturated oils like olive and canola can be used freely as long as you don't get carried away, because they are still high in calories.

Dairy Products: One cup of milk or yogurt is a normal serving size. Be sure to choose non-fat or low-fat products and watch out for added sugar. Cheese is a good source of protein but even low fat versions are high in saturated fat so use them sparingly. A serving should be about the size of your three middle fingers.

Portion sizes are an *estimate* of what your body needs. Start with the guidelines above but stop eating before you feel full. It takes a little time for your brain to know what's in your stomach and shut down the hunger signal. If you wait until you feel totally full before you stop eating, that delay can result in your eating more than you need to. You can always eat more if you are still hungry, but once you have overeaten there isn't much you can do about it.

ENERGY BALANCE

Just as important as how much you eat is the need to balance that amount of food with activity and exercise. This is called energy balance and it is critical to maintaining a healthy weight. There are other things besides energy balance which can affect your weight, but energy balance is the most important. Food energy is measured in calories. If the amount of energy or calories that you consume is greater than the amount of energy your body spends for metabolism and movement, you will gain weight. If you take in less energy than your body spends, you will lose weight. The more you eat, the more active you must be to offset the extra calories. It's that simple.

Understanding Energy Balance

Food energy is measured in calories
Energy Intake = Energy Spent → Maintain Body Weight
Energy Intake > Energy Spent → Weight Gain
Energy Intake < Energy Spent → Weight Loss

Energy Intake:
Carbohydrates   = 4 calories/gram
Proteins   = 4 calories/gram
Fats   = 9 calories/gram
Alcohol   = 7 calories/gram

Energy Expenditure
Metabolism or Basal Metabolic Rate (BMR): This is the amount of calories your body spends to perform all basic functions necessary to life. It is measured when you are at rest and is affected by age, sex, height and how much lean body mass you have.
Activity and Exercise: The extra calories you burn by moving your body. The more, faster, or harder you move, the more calories you burn.
Thermic Effect of Food: The calories your body spends to digest and metabolize food.
Adaptive Thermogenesis: The calories your body spends to adjust to changes in your environment and your health.

Carbohydrates, proteins, and fats all contain energy or calories as does alcohol. However it is a popular misconception that vitamins and minerals give you energy. These micronutrients play an important role in the processes that release energy from food, but they don't contain any energy of their own.

WHAT TO EAT

In addition to water, there are five types of nutrients that your body must have to create optimum health: carbohydrates, protein, fat, vitamins and minerals. These are the things that your body is made of and that it needs a constant supply of to remain in good working order. Research has also uncovered the importance of a group of compounds found in plants called phytochemicals that may play critical roles in your health as well. Each of these components is equally important. Without sufficient amounts of any of them, your health will suffer and your amazing body will not be able to operate at peak efficiency.

The source, packaging and combination of these nutrients is important because it determines how readily available they are and how well your body can utilize them. Always try to choose foods that are whole or as close to the way nature created them as possible. Whole food is preferable to processed food because it usually contains more nutrients. Take grains for example. When whole wheat flour is converted into white flour, vitamins, minerals, and fiber are all lost. In order to compensate for those losses, flour is usually "enriched." Enriching flour adds back some of the vitamins, but not the rest of the nutrients that were originally present in the whole grain. Processed foods are usually higher in salt and sugar than unprocessed foods, and they are more likely to contain additives such as artificial colors, flavoring, and preservatives. Manufacturers add these chemicals to food in order to make them more appealing or to have a longer shelf life, not because they are beneficial to the health of the consumer. Processed foods also tend to be more expensive even though they are less nutritious.

A whole food has only one ingredient, itself. It is minimally processed, if at all, and still contains most of its naturally occurring nutrients and no additives. Fruits, vegetables, grains, and meats from naturally raised animals fall under the definition of a whole food. The further you move away from "whole" the less nutritious a food can become. There are exceptions such as grinding seeds to make them more digestible, but overall, eating whole foods improves the nutrient quality of your diet.

CHOOSE ORGANIC FOODS WHENEVER YOU CAN

Buying organic foods is better for your body and for the earth. Organic foods are produced without the use of chemicals, pesticides or hormones. Once only available in health food stores, organic products have become very main stream and are now available in most large grocery chains. With the implementation of national standards, you can buy Certified Organic foods with confidence that you are getting what you pay for.

GOOD REASONS TO GO ORGANIC

- **More Nutritious:** Fruits and vegetables grown organically have significantly higher levels of cancer-fighting antioxidants than conventionally grown foods.
- **Better Taste:** Organic farming methods nourish the soil which in turn nourishes the plants and results in better tasting products. Many top chefs choose organic foods for just this reason.
- **Reduce Exposure to Toxic Chemicals:** Herbicides and pesticides are toxic chemicals designed to kill living organisms. Research to address concerns over their potential harmful affects on humans including birth defects, nerve damage and cancer has shown conflicting results but are known to be a concern for children. It is better to be safe than sorry.

- **Additive Free:** Organic foods don't contain additives such as preservatives, artificial colors and flavors.
- **Support Family Farming:** Because of increased demand for organic products, large producers are starting to make the conversion to organic practices, but most organic farms are small, family owned enterprises.
- **Protect Our Natural Resources:** Pesticides contaminate ground water, and conventional farming practices lead to depleted soil which requires increasing amounts of fertilizer to be productive. Organic farmers use natural methods of pest control and soil replenishment to keep the land fertile. These methods protect our water and help prevent soil erosion. They also reduce fossil fuel dependency and the release of greenhouse gasses into the atmosphere.

Organic food costs more than conventional food, but its health benefits and sustainable, ecologically sound production methods are cost effective in the long run.

THE IMPORTANCE OF VARIETY AND MODERATION

There is no one perfect food other than perhaps breast milk, and that is only perfect for infants. A given food may be an excellent source of one or several nutrients but notoriously lacking in another. Milk is a good source of protein and calcium, but a poor source of iron. Meat is an excellent source of iron, but a poor source of calcium, and neither meat nor milk contains any phytochemicals at all. In order to make sure that you get all the different nutrients that your body needs it is important to eat a variety of foods, not just stick with a few favorites. Many cuisines such as those of the Mediterranean and the Far East offer definite health benefits over typical

American fare. Sampling the cuisines of foreign lands is a fun way to explore interesting new flavors and food combinations, so be a little adventurous and broaden your dietary horizons.

Choosing a variety of foods is also important in helping you to minimize your exposure to the unhealthy constituents in food. Even the healthiest of foods carries some potential risks. Take liver for example. Liver is the nutrient processing center for the body. It is also the body's detoxification center. All of the blood leaving your gut goes directly to the liver where newly arriving nutrients are processed, and toxins, heavy metals and pesticides are cleansed from the blood before it continues on to more sensitive organs like the heart and the brain. The liver performs the same functions in animals, so while liver may be a concentrated source of vitamins and minerals, it is also a concentrated source of the unhealthy products that it removed from its owner's blood. Fruits and vegetables are extremely healthful, but they may also be a source of not so healthful herbicides, pesticides and fertilizer residues.

There are no good foods or bad foods, there are only foods that contain greater or lesser amounts of good and bad things. All foods can be part of a healthy diet as long as you consume them in moderation. The more bad stuff a food contains, the less of it you should eat, but you don't have to completely deprive yourself of foods you love if they aren't healthy choices. Eating a little bit of everything and not too much of anything is the way to go.

ENJOY YOUR FOOD

Food is one of the great pleasures in life. It is a sensory delight that can be appreciated in many ways if you take the time to enjoy it. The colors, textures and flavors of food offer a feast for your eyes as well as your palate, and the aromas of food can be intoxicating. Engaging all of your senses in your experience of food is good for your soul and good for your health. When you take the time to appreciate all aspects of a meal— how it looks, how it smells, the feel of it in your mouth, the subtle nuances of how the flavors blend—you eat less than when you wolf food down in a hurry. You also digest it better.

When you are rushed or upset your body experiences a mild version of something called the "fight or flight" response—an instinctive set of biological reactions designed to help you survive in emergency situations. In a true emergency, things like your heart beating faster and blood pressure rising improve your ability to defend yourself or escape the danger, but digestion does not, so your digestive tract basically shuts down until the crisis passes. In an emergency, this response may help keep you alive, but when it is caused by stress rather than danger, it can make it difficult to digest and metabolize your food.

In today's busy world it can sometimes be a challenge to find enough time to eat at all, much less enough time to sit and enjoy your meals in a calm and relaxed way, but there are a few simple things that you can do to that might be helpful. First, don't use meal time for discussing stressful issues. The time to confront a co-worker, argue over family finances, or scold a child isn't at the dinner table. Getting upset while you try to eat will not only impair digestion, but it can ruin your appetite and spoil the enjoyment of your meal. Try not to multi-task either. Paying attention to what you are eating will help you to appreciate your food and remain aware of how much you are eating. You are likely to eat far more if you are consuming food on autopilot rather than eating consciously. Whenever you can, take a few moments before you eat to close your eyes and take some deep breaths and relax. It will help to calm your system, prepare your body to accept the feast ahead, and increase your enjoyment of your food.

Eating isn't just about refueling your body, it's a centerpiece of life. Food is a medium for social interaction and religious ceremony. It's an integral part of every ritual from celebrations to peace offerings and it is meant to be enjoyed. Eating healthfully doesn't mean giving up the joy of food, it means learning to appreciate it in every way using all of your senses and making healthier choices. As you learned in the last section there are no good foods or bad foods. You are free to enjoy any food as long as you follow two simple rules:

1. **Always eat what you need before you eat what you want**
2. **Everything in moderation**

If you want a piece of pie, you can have a piece of pie, just make sure that before you do, you give your body everything it needs to be healthy *first*. If you have consumed enough water, fresh fruits and vegetables, high quality protein, whole grains and healthy fats, there won't be a lot of room left over and you will likely be satisfied with a small piece of pie instead of a large one. There's nothing wrong with indulging in something that has little or no nutritional value as long as you don't overdo it and it doesn't replace the healthy foods your body needs.

Denying yourself the foods you desire will make you feel deprived and encourage you to rebound, often dramatically. Having a little pie when you really want it is much better than eating a whole pie because you have missed it so much. No matter how long you live, life is too short to deny yourself the pleasures of food, and enjoying your food doesn't have to mean jeopardizing your health.

A Word about Alcohol

A glass of wine or a cocktail can help you to relax and add enjoyment to a meal. It's good for your heart and may help prevent you from having a stroke, but when it comes to alcohol consumption, moderation isn't just important, it's critical. A little alcohol provides health benefits, but just a little *too much* alcohol can have serious consequences. It contributes to liver disease, cancer (especially of the breast), disrupts your metabolism, and interferes with your sleep. It throws off the acid-base balance of your system and can damage the lining of your stomach. It impairs digestion making nutritional deficiencies more likely, and it's addictive, especially for those who have a family history of alcoholism. It impairs your judgment and can lead to engaging in risky behaviors. Drugs and alcohol are the number one cause of traffic related deaths.

Excess alcohol consumption can also cause you to gain weight. By disrupting normal metabolism, alcohol has been shown to reduce the body's use of fat for fuel by as much as 30%. It also contains 75% more calories per gram than do carbohydrates or protein. These extra calories together with the reduction in fat utilization can increase the amount of fat stored by your body. Alcoholic beverages that are high in carbohydrates compound this effect even further and can quickly lead to the development of the typical "beer belly" seen on heavy drinkers.

People who drink in moderation are generally healthier than people who don't drink at all, and certainly more so than those who drink too much, but just how much is moderation?

Generally, no more than one drink per day for women and older adults, and no more than two per day for men. And no, you can't save up all week and have a six pack on Saturday.

What Counts as One Drink?

12 ounces of beer
5 ounces of wine
1.5 ounces of 80 proof liquor

THE KEYS TO FEEDING YOUR BODY WELL

1. Drink enough water everyday.
2. Eat only when you are hungry and stop **before** you are full. ***Enough is better than more!***
3. Eat every three to four hours; start the day with a healthy breakfast and end it with a bedtime snack.
4. Balance how much you feed your body with how much you move your body.
5. Choose whole foods that are as close to the way nature made them as possible, and choose organic foods whenever you can.
6. Avoid additives including artificial colors, flavors and preservatives.
7. Eat lots of fruits and vegetables.
8. Always choose whole grains and limit your intake of sugar, corn syrup, breads, pasta and snacks.
9. Eat more nuts, beans, soy, seafood and poultry, and less red meat.
10. Avoid trans fatty acids, saturated fat and fried foods.
11. Always try to eat balanced meals and snacks that contain carbohydrate, protein and fat.
12. Remember variety and moderation. Eat a little of everything and not too much of anything.
13. Enjoy your food but eat what you *need* before you eat what you *want*.
14. Avoid eating too much salt or drinking too much alcohol.
15. Use dietary supplements as insurance, not as a replacement for healthy eating.

2

LET THE FLUIDS FLOW!

In your car, fluids are used to keep your engine cool, wash your windshield, lubricate all of the moving parts, and keep the pressure constant in the hydraulic systems. Without enough fluids the engine would overheat, you wouldn't be able to see where you were going, your wheels wouldn't turn, and you would have to work a lot harder to steer and stop. Basically, without enough of the right kinds of fluids, nothing in your car would work very well.

Without enough fluids, your body doesn't work very well either. Even a small drop in your body's water level can give you a headache and make it difficult to concentrate. It can cause constipation, make you feel tired or weak, increase your risk of injury, and dry out your skin. Dehydration thickens your blood, increasing your risk of having a heart attack, and over time chronic dehydration can increase your risk of developing kidney stones and bladder cancer. Not drinking enough water can even fool you into thinking that you are hungry when all you really need is a drink! Drinking enough water is critical because of all the unique roles it plays in maintaining your health and vitality.

Water makes up about 60% of your body's weight and it is involved in every bodily function. It delivers vital nutrients to your cells, carries away their wastes, and helps to flush the body of toxins. If you are not properly hydrated, your cells will not be as well nourished and waste products can build up in your system.

Water is also your body's shock absorber. It provides cushioning for everything from your knees to your brain and spinal cord, and along with fat, helps protect your organs from bruising when you drive on bumpy roads. Body fluids provide lubrication which reduces the wear and tear on your joints, makes it easier to swallow, and keeps your eyes comfortable. As an essential component of your body's cooling system, it keeps the rest of you comfortable as well.

Your body is producing heat at all times via metabolism and physical activity and it depends on perspiration to rid itself of any excess. As water evaporates from your skin, it takes body heat with it, helping to prevent you from becoming overheated. Without sufficient water in the system, heat exhaustion, heat cramps and heat stroke—a life threatening condition—can set in more quickly. Since sweating causes you to lose more water, the more you sweat the more water that you must replace. Sweating also helps to rid your body and skin of toxins.

If you are a fitness fanatic, a weekend warrior, or just trying to get in shape, being properly hydrated is critical not only to prevent heat related problems, but also to help you play your best. Just a 3% drop in your body's water level impairs your muscles' ability to do work. That means you won't be as strong, your endurance will be reduced, and so will your overall ability to perform on the course, the field, the court, or in the gym. Under some conditions, you can lose up to a quart an hour of fluids during strenuous exercise.

You can't count on thirst to guide you in drinking enough fluids. Thirst often lags behind your need for water, especially in children, the elderly, and during exercise. This gap is even more dramatic in hot, humid weather. By the time you feel thirsty you are already dehydrated. To make sure that your body is getting as much fluid as it needs, make drinking water a routine part of your every day activities. Carry a water bottle with you and sip on it throughout the day. Drinking a large glass of water before each meal will not only help to increase your fluid intake but will also make you feel full sooner and help you to eat less.

So how much water do you actually have to drink to stay healthy? Eight glasses a day has been the standard recommendation for a long time, but it is a general estimate at best. How much water you need every day depends on many variables including how much and what kinds of foods you eat. Diets high in protein or sodium or low in calories increase your need for water, as does a high fiber diet (but high fiber is a *good* thing).

Your water needs are also affected by your age, your environment, your activity level, medications you may be taking, and a host of other considerations. Therefore, the best advice is to drink frequently throughout the day, especially before, during, and after exercise, and check the color of your urine. It should be a pale straw color or even colorless. If it's darker, like the color of apple juice, then your body is in need of more fluids. If it's a bright yellow or fluorescent orange, it probably means that you are taking more dietary supplements than what your body can use and the excess is being disposed of via your kidneys, and yes, that requires more water too. If you need a specific number to aim for in order to feel comfortable that you are getting enough fluids, eight cups per day is an acceptable place to begin, but depending on your body and other factors, it may not be enough.

WATER SOURCES

Water should be your beverage of choice whether it comes from a bottle or a tap, is filtered or unfiltered. Unlike soft drinks or coffee, it doesn't contain calories or caffeine, rob your bones of calcium, or turn your teeth yellow. If water doesn't appeal to you, there are lots of alternative drinks that can help you get enough fluids each day. At the top of the list—herbal teas—they count about equal to water when it comes to hydration. Green tea and black tea are also good choices for increasing your water intake because they provide healthful antioxidants. Unlike herbal teas, green and black tea contain some caffeine, a diuretic which causes you to lose some of the water you consume, but not enough to be a problem. Coffee contains more caffeine than tea so it too causes you to lose some water, but not as much as we used to think. For each cup of coffee you consume, you can count about 50% of it towards your daily water needs.

Tea: A Very Healthful Choice!

The health effects of green tea have been studied extensively and the benefits of this beverage are impressive. An excellent source of antioxidants, green tea has been linked to lower heart disease and cancer risk, and the prevention of osteoporosis. It can also fight viruses and inhibit the growth of bacteria that cause illness, dental caries and bad breath. To reap the benefits of tea, allow it to steep for several minutes before drinking.

Pure fruit juice is a good choice because it provides water along with vitamins and minerals, but remember that it is high is sugar and calories so don't overdo it. Try not to drink more than 8 ounces per day and make sure that what you are drinking is 100% juice and isn't a "juice beverage" containing large amounts of corn syrup or other sweeteners. For a refreshing change and to cut the calories and sugar, add plain seltzer to your juice and top it off with a twist of fresh lemon or lime.

Milk and soy milk contain a high percentage of water plus protein, carbohydrates, fat, vitamins, and minerals, so they are good choices as well, but like fruit juice, they contain calories that you may or may not want. Also like juice, they are not absorbed as quickly, so if you are really thirsty, head for the water first.

Soft drinks can be counted as being about 50% water, but they are not a good choice at all. Most contain anywhere from 6 to 10 teaspoons of sugar per serving—that's like adding 6 to 10 packets of sugar to each cup of your coffee or tea. Most also contain artificial colors, flavors, preservatives, and other additives that are better avoided. Some also contain caffeine. Soft drinks designed specifically for hydration such as sports drinks may have advantages for serious athletes or if you exercise in hot, humid conditions, but many still contain high levels of sugar and additives.

What About Carbonation?

Carbonation comes from dissolving carbon dioxide (CO_2) in water. It is quickly absorbed in the gastrointestinal tract and is carried to the lungs for exhalation. Your body produces lots of CO_2 as a result of normal energy production and it is well equipped to efficiently remove it from your blood. CO_2 doesn't affect bone health, but phosphoric acid (phosphate) which is contained in some carbonated beverages can increase calcium losses.

Alcohol is a poor choice for hydration because of its diuretic effect. In fact, for every beer, glass of wine or cocktail that you consume, you should drink an extra glass of water just to offset your losses. Alternating drinks containing alcohol with a glass of water will help you to drink in moderation, and if you should have "one too many," it can help reduce some of the classic symptoms of a hang over like headache and weakness—both side effects of dehydration.

Healthful Hint
Drink lots of water and avoid alcohol when you fly. The dry, recycled air in an aircraft can dry out your nasal passages making you more susceptible to infection from airborne germs.

BOTTLED WATER VS. TAP WATER

Bottled water is the fastest growing segment of the beverage market. Americans spent over $7 billion dollars in the year 2002 on plain waters, sparkling waters, spring waters, designer waters and water from municipal supplies dressed up with fancy labels posing as designer water. When it comes to whether you should buy your water in a bottle, or fill your own bottle from the faucet in your kitchen, it's mostly a matter of taste and convenience.

Bottled water must meet the same safety standards as municipal-system water and the sources from which it is derived are just as vulnerable to contamination as the sources of tap water are. In fact many brands of bottled water *are* tap water. An inspiring picture of pristine mountains or a lovely glacier on the outside of the bottle doesn't mean that's where the water inside the bottle came from, guarantee its safety, or make it healthier. Bottled water isn't healthier for the environment either. It uses lots of energy to manufacture, fill and transport the bottles. If you are going to purchase bottled water, be sure to recycle your empty containers.

Why Buy Bottled Water?

Taste: If you don't like the taste of the local tap water, bottled water offers a pleasant alternative. It comes in many varieties, with and without flavoring agents added.

Health: Many people believe that bottled water is better for you than tap water. Some bottled waters are processed or filtered more than tap water to remove impurities, but not all are. If you prefer filtered water, simple home filtering systems are readily available. Some bottled waters contain additives such as vitamins and minerals, but for basic hydration, these offer no special health benefits. In fact "waters" which contain sweeteners, stimulants like caffeine, preservatives and other additives may actually be less healthy for you. There are also concerns about traces of harmful chemicals leaching from plastic containers into the water, especially if they are exposed to excessive heat like that found inside of your car on a hot summer day. If the water in your area or your home is contaminated for some reason, using bottled water is a good choice.

Convenience: Available in a variety of sizes, water bottles are easy to pack and take with you wherever you go and are readily available in most locations. However, you pay quite a premium for this convenience. Tap water costs less than a penny a gallon, while bottled waters usually cost $1.20 or more for 12 ounces—that's more than 600 times the price of tap water! If you are on a budget, fill your own bottle and take it with you.

Image: Some people drink bottled waters to project a certain image of themselves. It's a way to let others know that they are health conscious or sophisticated. Carrying a water bottle wherever you go is a healthy choice that has also become a chic thing to do.

Whatever your reason for choosing bottled water, it's important to know what you are getting. Here's a quick rundown on the different types of bottled water:

Spring water is a type of groundwater that has risen from an underground source to the earth's surface. Like all groundwater, spring water can be contaminated by farming practices or industry, so the location of the spring is very important. Spring water may or may not be carbonated, may or may not be called mineral water, and may or may not be processed. If it is labeled "Natural" it is not processed in any way before bottling.

Mineral water is simply water that contains minerals. All water except distilled water contains minerals, but most bottled mineral water comes from springs. If it is labeled "Natural" no additional minerals have been added to it.

Distilled water is water that has been evaporated into steam then recondensed leaving many impurities and all solid matter behind, but it still may contain some organic chemicals. Because minerals give water much of its flavor, distilled water usually has little taste.

Sparkling water contains carbonation or gaseous bubbles. The gases can be naturally occurring or added. Many sparkling waters are high in sodium.

Seltzer water contains carbonation but no minerals or salts have been added. True seltzers may contain the "essence" of fruit adding extra flavor but no calories, sugar or salts, but read labels carefully. Some beverages calling themselves "seltzers" actually contain sweeteners such as corn syrup (which adds calories), artificial ingredients, and salts.

Enhanced waters may contain anything from corn syrup to caffeine. They are usually filtered tap water with minerals, flavorings, herbs or stimulants added to improve taste and or enhance performance in some way. Like the seltzers, some also contain calories, sweeteners, salts and other ingredients.

Unless you are a serious athlete who might need more than just water for proper hydration and improved performance, or you exercise in hot humid weather, the healthiest choice is plain, simple water. If a pleasant flavor will help you to drink

more, flavored seltzers that contain no added salt or preservatives, and enhanced waters that don't contain sweeteners or
artificial ingredients are also excellent choices. It's best to avoid
products that call themselves water but contain things your
body doesn't need.

3

TO CARB OR NOT TO CARB?

Carbohydrates are an important part of any healthy diet. They are an essential source of fuel, especially for your brain and central nervous system, and they are required for the efficient burning of another fuel, fat. They may reduce your risk of heart disease by lowering your cholesterol, and they keep your gastrointestinal tract moving smoothly which helps to prevent constipation and hemorrhoids, and reduces your risk of developing colon cancer. But all carbohydrates are not created equal. The *kind* of carbohydrates that you include in your diet makes all the difference in whether they contribute to your health or not.

Except for those found in milk and dairy products, all carbohydrates come from plants. Using radiant energy from the sun, plants are able to convert water and carbon dioxide into sugars to use as energy or fuel. They can also store this energy for future use as starch.

Healthy carbohydrates are the ones that are still in the natural package in which nature created them, and those that do not cause your blood sugar to rise too rapidly after you consume them. Fruits and vegetables contain simple sugars as well as complex carbohydrates and they are some of the healthiest foods you can eat. In addition to the fuel they contain, they also provide fiber to keep you regular, vitamins, minerals, extra water and phytochemicals,—those amazing plant based compounds that we are only now realizing the importance of. Whole grains such as whole wheat, old fashioned oatmeal or steel cut oats, and brown rice offer the same advantages. All of these foods are what we call **nutrient dense**. Nutrient dense means you get a lot of nutrition per calorie. It's like getting a lot of value for your money. Because they are high in fiber and may contain some fat, the sugars they contain enter your bloodstream gradually in a way that your body can handle very well.

Refined carbohydrates are those that have been removed from their original packaging, like table sugar, corn syrup and white flour. These refined carbohydrates and the foods made from them like sweets, soft drinks, breads, and pasta, contain lots of empty calories. Even though white flour is usually enriched, the enrichment process only adds back a small amount of the nutrients that are lost in refining. These carbohydrates are no longer in the natural form that your body was designed to use them in. As a result, they can easily overload your body's fuel management system causing you to feel miserable, gain weight, and have an increased risk of diabetes and heart disease, especially if they are consumed alone or in large quantities.

Since having enough glucose (the simple sugar every cell in your body depends on for fuel) available for cellular activity is critical to your health and survival, your body goes to great lengths to maintain the proper level of it in your blood. When your blood sugar level falls, it is known as hypoglycemia. Hypoglycemia makes you feel tired, weak and irritable. You may even become dizzy or shaky.

Note: Blood glucose levels between 65 and 115 mg/dL are considered normal, but for some individuals, their "comfort zone" is narrower and they experience the discomforts associated with low blood sugar even though clinically, their levels are within the normal range.

To correct the problem, your cells send a message to your brain letting it know that they are getting low on fuel, and your brain in turn lets you know that it's time to refill your tank by making you hungry. After you eat, your blood sugar level begins to rise, you feel better, and your appetite diminishes. The increased sugar in your blood causes your pancreas to release the hormone insulin which acts like a key that unlocks the door of your cells to allow the glucose in. As the cells continue to withdraw sugar from your blood, your blood glucose level starts to fall and the whole process begins again. That's how it's *supposed* to work. But when you consume too many or the wrong kind of carbohydrates a lot can go wrong with this system.

If your blood sugar rises too high, your pancreas is forced to respond by producing more insulin to bring it under control. If for some reason your pancreas can't respond and your blood sugar remains elevated, it becomes a condition known as hyperglycemia. Chronic hyperglycemia is known as diabetes. If your blood sugar rises too quickly, it can cause your pancreas to over-react and produce too much insulin. This extra insulin in turn can cause a rapid fall in your blood sugar level causing hypoglycemia along with its unpleasant symptoms, and making you feel hungry when you really don't need more food. Instead of the gradual rise and fall of blood sugar that should occur, you have severe peaks and valleys, both of which are bad for your health.

NORMAL AND SPIKING BLOOD SUGAR RESPONSES

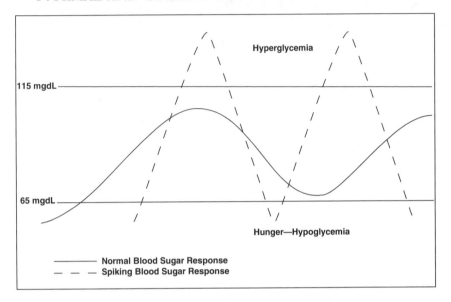

When there is more sugar in the system at one time than your cells can use (a peak), the excess is collected by your liver and converted to fat. This can cause an increase in your triglyceride levels—a risk factor for heart disease—as well as increasing your chances of becoming overweight, another risk factor for heart disease. Sugar can easily be converted to fat, but fat cannot be converted to sugar. When your blood sugar falls too low, you must consume more carbohydrates to replenish it. If you regularly choose refined carbohydrates, you will likely trigger the same negative cycle to be repeated over and over again with all of the excess calories being converted to fat. However, if you choose non-refined carbohydrates which cause your blood sugar to rise gradually, or a well balanced meal that includes protein and fat along with your carbohydrates, you can interrupt the cycle. If you don't interrupt the cycle, your fuel management system can become even more disrupted.

As your percentage of body fat increases, your cells become

more resistant to insulin—the key no longer quite fits the lock—and your pancreas pumps out even more insulin in an attempt to overcome the resistance. This exaggerates an already bad situation and can eventually lead to the pancreas wearing out and not being able to produce enough insulin to meet your needs. Obesity is an important contributing factor to diabetes. The more overweight you become the less your body is able to manage carbohydrates effectively and the easier it becomes to gain even more weight, a very negative downward spiral.

So why not simply stop eating carbohydrates altogether? Because you would miss out on all of the health benefits of carbohydrates mentioned earlier, and your body wouldn't run well.

Your brain and central nervous system *require* glucose for fuel. They simply can't live without it. If there were no glucose available, they would cease to function and you would die. Fat can't be converted to glucose, but protein can, so when you don't consume enough carbohydrates, your body starts borrowing protein from your blood, organs and muscles to meet it's sugar needs. Instead of using protein for building and repairing tissue, your body uses it for fuel and creates waste products in the process that your liver and kidneys must deal with. One of these waste products, uric acid, increases your risk for developing painful kidney stones. If you have enough carbohydrates in your diet, it spares your protein for more important uses.

Glucose is also required to burn fat efficiently and completely. Glucose acts like kindling and oxygen. Like kindling it helps to get the fire started and burning hot enough so that you can add larger logs—the fat. Like oxygen, it provides the ingredients necessary for the logs (fat) to burn entirely. When there isn't enough glucose available, your body can't metabolizes fat normally so it uses a different metabolic pathway which produces something called ketones. When denied glucose your brain can adapt by using these ketones to meet some of its energy requirements, but it cannot use them to completely replace glucose. Because ketones are acidic, your body must take steps to neutralize this acid or it can disturb the normal pH balance of your system and do serious damage to your organs. Ketosis causes you to lose lots of water which is part of the reason why people on extremely low carbohydrate diets lose weight rapidly during the first few weeks. Seeing quick results may be very inspiring and provide the incentive to keep losing weight, but long term ketosis is not healthy. No diet, not even the very carbohydrate restrictive ones recommend avoiding all carbohydrates long term.

The question really isn't whether or not to eat carbohydrates, but rather which ones to eat and when. And the answer is quite simple. Intact, unrefined carbohydrates that are still in the package nature created them in are good choices and refined carbohydrates that have been separated from their packaging should be considered a treat and consumed in small quantities or not at all. There are only a few exceptions to this rule and those are intact foods that produce a high glycemic load such as potatoes.

How high and how fast blood sugar rises on average in response to a certain food is called that food's glycemic index. When you multiply that index by the number of grams of carbohydrate found in a serving, it gives you the foods glycemic load; a number that reflects that food's impact on your blood glucose and insulin levels—the higher the number, the greater the impact. The glycemic load of a food is affected by how much the food has been processed and by how much fiber and fat it contains. The more it has been processed, the higher its glycemic load. Drinking orange juice produces a higher glycemic load than eating an orange because processing has both reduced the amount of fiber, and the sugars are more readily available. Finely grinding grains also makes the carbohydrates easier and faster to digest. Even if the whole grain is used, fine grinding will raise the glycemic load of the resulting flour. A cup of white rice and a cup of beans have about the same amount of carbohydrate but because the beans contain lots of fiber and white rice contains almost none, the glycemic load of the rice is almost three times that of the beans.

The glycemic load of a food can be tempered by what you consume with it. If you eat a high glycemic load food but combine it with other foods high in fiber or fat, it will slow down the digestion of the carbohydrates. For instance, if you are going to have a slice of white bread instead of whole wheat bread, you can lower the impact of the bread by topping it with crunchy peanut butter which contains fat, fiber and some protein. Of course peanut butter on whole wheat bread would be a better choice, but if white bread is the only option available, you can eat it in a healthier way by combining it with other nutritious, slower digesting foods. Dairy products including milk are the only non-plant source of carbohydrates. Dairy products also contain protein and possibly some fat, which slows the absorption of the sugar they contain known as lactose. Some individuals lack the necessary enzyme to digest this sugar and it can cause abdominal bloating and cramping. If you are lactose intolerant you can purchase reduced lactose products or take the enzyme in pill form to help you digest dairy products.

FIBER IS FABULOUS

Carbohydrates that can't be digested by your body are called fiber (also known as roughage) and they come in two forms: soluble and insoluble. Soluble fibers such as oat bran help to lower the level of cholesterol in your body, and insoluble fibers like wheat bran help to keep your stools soft and easy to pass. They also provide an aerobic workout for your digestive tract. Fiber stimulates the muscles of your intestines and colon to contract and become more toned. This reduces your risk of developing diverticulosis; a condition that occurs when the intestinal walls become weak and bulge out in places. Additional benefits of fiber:

- Absorbs water and swells, helping you to feel full longer and eat less.
- Helps prevent sudden rises in blood sugar levels by slowing the digestion and absorption of carbohydrates.
- High fiber diets are associated with a reduced risk of colon cancer.

You should try to consume between 25–30 grams of fiber each day. If you are choosing most of your carbohydrates from the "Best Choices" list, this will occur naturally. If not, you might consider adding a tablespoon or so of bran to your morning cereal. Fiber supplements are fine, but getting your fiber from your food is best. If you haven't been eating much fiber, add it to your diet slowly to avoid excess gas and discomfort. Your body needs time to adjust, even to healthy choices!

ARTIFICIAL SWEETENERS

Artificial sweeteners are just that, artificial. If you need to sweeten your food or beverages to make them more appealing, use the natural herb Stevia. Available in natural food stores as a dietary supplement, stevia is extremely sweet and only very small amounts of it are needed to flavor beverages or foods. I strongly suggest that you also avoid foods and beverages made with artificial sweeteners.

BEST CARBOHYDRATE CHOICES

These sources of carbohydrates are extremely healthful and nutrient packed. They should make up a large part of your overall diet.

- Vegetables except potatoes, cassava and starchy roots
- Fruits
- Whole grains including whole wheat, whole oats, rye, barley, quinoa, bulgur, kasha and brown rice
- Products made with whole grains including whole wheat or whole grain bread and tortillas, whole wheat pasta, whole wheat pancakes, muffins and whole grain breakfast cereals
- Beans and legumes

OCCASIONALLY ACCEPTABLE CHOICES

Far more refined than the best choices, these foods consumed alone will raise your blood sugar levels quickly and only provide modest amounts of nutrients. To reduce their impact on your blood sugar level, eat them as part of a balanced meal that also includes a source of protein and healthful fats. If you are overweight or not very active you should eat these sparingly. If you are lean or very active you can consume a little more of them.

- Pasta
- Breads which contain only some or no whole grains including bagels,muffins, pancakes and waffles
- Breakfast cereals that contain only some or no whole grains
- Potatoes, cassava and starchy roots

FOR SPECIAL OCCASIONS ONLY

These foods have very little if any nutritional value and will raise your blood sugar quickly. They should be consumed only after you have given your body everything it needs first, and only infrequently. They shouldn't be part of your daily diet.

- Candy
- Cakes, cookies, pastry, donuts, and other sweet baked goods
- Processed foods that are high in carbohydrates
- Sweetened soft drinks
- Snack foods including chips, crackers, pretzels etc. Even if they are made with whole grains, these foods are usually high in salt and possibly trans fatty acids as well.

Know What You Are Buying

Ingredients are listed in descending order by weight. The first ingredients listed are the most plentiful and the ingredients that are present in the smallest amounts are listed towards the end. Always look for the words "**whole** wheat" or "**whole** grain" at the beginning of the list. If the word "whole" is listed farther down, you are getting mainly refined grains. "Enriched" or "fortified" means nutrients have been added, but it is still refined. Many breads use colorful terms to imply that they are healthier, but most mean nothing nutritionally. If it doesn't say "whole", it isn't whole! The only way to know for sure is to read the ingredient list.

4

PROTEIN'S PROPER PLACE

The word protein is derived from the Greek word proteios meaning "of prime importance," and important it is—but no more so than any of the other essential components of a healthy diet. If you tried to live on protein alone you would have a very short life, because proteins don't work alone. The perception that protein is the most important element in a healthy diet has led to the misconception that you need a lot of it to be healthy and the more you consume the better. As with most nutrients, *enough is better than more!* Excess protein, just like excess carbohydrate or excess fat will be converted to body fat, and it can have other negative consequences as well. High protein and low protein diets have their place in medicine, but for creating and maintaining a healthy body, *adequate* amounts of protein are what you need. Most American diets are more than adequate when it comes to protein.

Proteins are used to create the structures of your body such as muscles, organs, tissues and cells. They are the building blocks of body chemicals such as hormones and enzymes, and they are the vehicles of the body's transportation system carrying oxygen and other materials to and from the cells. Your body can store lots of fat and some carbohydrate, but it doesn't store proteins. In order to have all the high quality protein you need to keep everything in your body running smoothly, you need to re-supply it daily.

All proteins are made up of smaller units called amino acids. How these individual units are combined determines the nature and use of the protein. Your body can make some of these amino acids if it has the raw materials to do so, but others must be consumed in your diet; these are the essential amino acids. When a protein source contains all of the essential amino acids in one place and it is digestible by humans, it is considered to be a complete protein. If one or more of the *essential* amino acids is missing, it is an incomplete protein. Most animal sources of protein such as meat, poultry, eggs, seafood, and milk are complete, but not all vegetable sources are. However, vegetable proteins complement each other. By simply eating a variety of foods, vegetarians are just as able to get all of the essential amino acids they need as are meat eaters.

Different sources of protein have different advantages. Vegetable sources, especially soy, are becoming more and more popular because they offer several health benefits over animal sources. They don't contain saturated fat and cholesterol, and growth hormones and antibiotics are not used in their production. They *do* contain fiber which can lower your cholesterol. Research has shown that regular consumption of soy protein in particular can reduce your risk of heart disease and may also be beneficial in reducing your risk of breast and prostrate cancer, osteoporosis, and in helping to reduce the symptoms of menopause.

In addition to being good for your body, replacing some of the animal protein in your diet with vegetable alternatives is also good for the earth. Raising animals to meet the world's protein needs uses up an incredible amount of resources and creates lots of pollution. It takes 12 pounds of grain, one gallon of gas, and 2,500 gallons of water to produce 1 pound of beef. Cattle ranching has encouraged the destruction of millions of acres of precious rain forest which contributes to changing weather patterns and global warming. The total volume of animal manure and the inappropriate disposal of it have led to issues of water and land contamination. According to the United Nations Food and Agriculture Organization, over 70% of fish stocks are fully exploited, overexploited, depleted or recovering from depletion.

Our land and our oceans are both exhaustible resources and the most powerful tool we possess to affect change is how we spend our money. By buying and eating less animal protein and more vegetable protein, we improve our health directly through the health benefits of consuming plant foods, and indirectly by contributing to a healthier, less polluted environment in which to live.

Just as protein doesn't stand alone in your body, neither does it stand alone in animals. Wherever you find protein you find other things as well, both good and bad. When you consume fatty, cold water fish, you get wonderfully healthful Omega-3 fatty acids which will be discussed in detail in the next chapter. Unfortunately, fish can also contain elevated levels of pesticides that have washed into our waters from agriculture and industry, along with mercury and other toxins. Meat is an excellent source of iron and zinc but it also contains saturated fat and cholesterol. Dairy products provide calcium but they too can be high in saturated fat. Choosing a variety of foods to meet your protein needs is the best way to strike a balance between getting what you need and avoiding what you don't.

How you prepare your food can also impact how healthful

your protein sources are. For example, it is better to buy lean cuts of meat than fatty ones, and broiling or grilling is better than frying.

Note: It is important to cook meat products sufficiently to destroy harmful microorganisms, but overcooking can lead to the production of carcinogenic chemicals, so don't eat charred or burned meats.

Removing the skin and visible fat from poultry means less saturated fat and less calories. Purchasing fat free or reduced fat dairy products can also cut out unwanted saturated fat.

Nuts are an excellent source of protein even though they are high in fat. The fats they contain are unsaturated so they don't raise your risk of heart disease. In fact just the opposite is true. Regular consumption of nuts has been shown to reduce the risk of heart disease in some people. The fat they contain can help you to feel full longer, and eat less too; just don't get carried away. A small handful of nuts in your salad or instead of another less healthful snack is great, but a small handful of nuts *in addition* to your regular foods and snacks each day can cause you to gain an extra 10 pounds in a year.

Regardless of which protein sources you choose, it is important to get the right amount. For every 10 pounds you weigh, you need to eat about 5 grams (g) of protein each day. If you are sedentary you will need a little less, if you are an athlete, you will need a little more, but for the average, active adult following the fitness recommendations in this manual, 5g is a good average. That means that if you weigh 120 pounds you need to eat about 60g of protein each day. If you weigh 180 pounds, you need to eat about 90g of protein each day. A four ounce serving of meat, fish or chicken contains about 30g of protein as does

1 cup of soybeans or miso and 1.5 cups of tofu. As you can see, two or three average servings per day will easily meet most people's needs. As always, let your body be your guide.

Extra protein doesn't help you build muscle any faster, only exercise can do that, but extra protein can cause your bones to lose more calcium. If you eat more protein, be sure to include more calcium in your diet as well to offset any losses and to drink extra fluids to help your kidneys handle the waste products safely.

5

FAT: FRIEND AND FOE

At eighty six years old my mother is still in excellent health. She's having some trouble with her eyes, and a recent car accident has caused her some setbacks, but unlike most people her age, she doesn't need to take any medications and she is still very active. She cuts her own lawn, shovels her own snow, and trims her own hedges. She also walks to church every day to make sure she gets her exercise, to interact with friends and to pray. Her diet is simple. She drinks tea several times a day, eats lots of vegetables, some grains, some poultry and fish and no red meat, and her motto has always been "Everything in moderation," including fats—and it's hard to argue with her success.

I was a student of nutrition in the seventies when the low fat recommendations where first being hammered home in an effort to reduce the incidence of heart disease, and it was always a source of contention between my mother and me. Regardless of the research I presented her with, she firmly believed that a little extra fat wasn't going to kill you and that too much "starch" as she called it, was going to make you fat. She also didn't believe in margarine. Thirty years later, it's turning out that she was right all along.

After decades of being slandered as the bad guy in nutrition, fat is making a comeback, not because the original information that started the low fat craze was wrong, but because it was incomplete. Nutrition is a relatively young science and whenever we hear advice on what to eat and what not to eat, it should always carry the footnote "To the best of our current knowledge." Sometimes new studies are so compelling that we act on their results quickly, but as research continues, our understanding of the complex issues and interrelationships between food and health deepens, and recommendations are adjusted to reflect that better understanding. When it comes to fat, what we understand now is that you can't lump them all together when trying to decide if they are good for you or bad for you.

Some fats like saturated fat found in red meat and trans fatty acids found in commercial baked goods, salad dressings and fried foods are very bad for you. Others like monounsaturated fat which is found in olive and canola oil, are very good for you. Some polyunsaturated fats are good for you as long as you don't eat too much of them. The key to fat and health is the same as the key to good nutrition in general—making sure you get enough of what you need and avoiding what you don't.

Fats are important components of several body structures. Your brain is built largely out of fat and so is the protective sheath that covers it and your spinal cord. The fat that surrounds your organs and lines the soles of your feet acts like a shock absorber padding them to prevent bruising and injury. Because fat repels water, it is an integral part of your cell membranes. Without fat, you would be one big bag of water rather than a collection of millions of individual cells. It insulates your body helping to keep you warm, and helps to keep your skin, hair and nails healthy. It is essential to manufacturing important body compounds such as hormones, and it stands in reserve to supply your body with energy whenever you need it.

Your body has a very limited capacity to store carbohydrates and it doesn't store excess protein for fuel at all. Fat contains more than twice the calories per gram as do carbohydrates or proteins, and it isn't bound with water so you can store a lot of energy in a much smaller amount of space. The unique chemical structure of fat allows your body to store an almost unlimited amount of it. If you are overweight you might not think this sounds like a good thing, but the ability to store energy is what enabled your ancestors to stay alive when the food supply wasn't as secure as it is today. In times of famine, natural disaster, and war, thin people were not as likely to survive as those who had a larger reserve of energy. This survival mechanism, like several others mentioned throughout this manual, hasn't adapted to our modern society where food is so plentiful and exercise is not. It doesn't have a built in circuit breaker to prevent overload. Nowadays instead of helping you to survive, your body's ability to store endless amounts of fat can contribute to the development of many diseases such as diabetes and heart disease.

Eating fat doesn't make you fat any more than eating carbohydrates makes you fat. Eating more food than your body needs to meet its energy needs is what makes you fat. If you eat more protein than your body can use, your body stores it as fat. If you eat more carbohydrate than your body can use, your body stores it as fat. If you eat more fat than you can use, it too gets stored as fat. Because fat contains more calories than protein or carbohydrate, foods that are high in fat also tend to be high in calories, but simply removing the fat and replacing the calories with carbohydrates doesn't make that food any less likely to contribute to weight gain. If it contains calories that your body doesn't need, a low fat or fat free cookie will still cause you to gain weight. If it causes your triglycerides to become elevated or contains trans fatty acids it won't be any better for your heart either.

Cutting back on fat is one way to reduce the total amount of calories that you are eating, but it's important to cut back on the right kind of fats rather than on all fats. Cutting back on fat indiscriminately deprives your body of valuable nutrients, important health benefits, and many of the pleasures of food. Fat carries both flavor and aroma and gives food that smooth feeling in your mouth. When you remove the fat from food you remove some of its appetite appeal as well. In order to overcome this, food manufacturers often replace fats with carbohydrates, additives and extra salt to make their low fat products palatable, but it doesn't make them healthier.

The best approach to fat is to reduce the amount of unhealthy fats you consume and make sure you consume enough of the healthy ones.

THE HEALTHY FAT CONTINUUM

Unhealthy   Healthy

◄---►

Trans Saturated   Polyunsaturated   Monounsaturated   Omega-3

The fats that seem to have the most negative effect on your health are trans fatty acids and saturated fats. Those with the most positive effect are omega-3 fatty acids and monounsaturated fats. But what exactly are these fats and where are they found?

All fats are made up of fatty acids, long chains of carbon atoms with hydrogen atoms bonded to them. If each carbon in the chain has all of the hydrogen atoms it can hold attached to it, and it can't hold anymore, then just like a sponge that can't hold any more water, it is saturated. The more chains of fully bonded carbons a fat contains, the more saturated it is and the more solid it will be at room temperature. Highly saturated fats are usually found in dairy and meat products. Palm and coconut are the only two vegetable oils that are high in saturated fats. Saturated fats raise the level of bad cholesterol in your blood, increasing your risk of heart disease, so they should be avoided as much as possible.

If one of the carbons in the chain is missing a hydrogen atom, then that fatty acid is *mono* (meaning one) unsaturated. If it has more than one missing, it is polyunsaturated. Unsaturated fats are liquid at room temperature and are mainly found in plant oils. Olive and canola oil, avocados and nuts are excellent sources of monounsaturated fat, while corn, soybean and safflower oils are good sources of *poly*unsaturated fat. Both are better for your heart, but too much polyunsaturated fat may increase your risk of cancer or displace the more valuable monounsaturated fats, which is why it's lower down on the healthy fat continuum. Olive oil is the cornerstone of the Mediterranean Diet and it can be used in place of butter or margarine for most purposes. Instead of butter, many Italian restaurants serve olive oil with fresh ground pepper for dipping bread. It makes a tasty salad dressing and can be used for cooking as well.

When Only Butter Will Do

To get the flavor of butter but control how much is used, peel back the wrapping on a stick of butter and use it like a crayon to "color" a cool pan before adding food. "Coloring" your toast instead of trying to evenly spread a pat of butter will also help you to get a little butter on each bite without using too much.

The two extremes on the continuum, trans fatty acids and omega-3 fatty acids are worth taking special note of. A very small amount of trans fatty acids occur in nature; the large majority of them are the result of a process called partial hydrogenation. Invented about a hundred years ago, partial hydrogenation involves forcing hydrogen atoms into unsaturated fats; in essence *trans-* forming them into more saturated ones. This process changes certain characteristics of the oil making it more practical for commercial use, but also produces some fatty acids that can be damaging to your health.

Unsaturated fats are more susceptible to oxidation than are saturated ones so they become rancid more quickly. Partial hydrogenation slows down this process so the oil and the products made with it can be stored for longer periods of time. Since these semi-solid fats and shortenings can also be used for baking, they are frequently found in commercial baked goods such as cookies, crackers and cakes. The longer an item can remain on the shelf without going stale, the less expensive it is to sell, which makes partially hydrogenated oils very attractive to food manufacturers.

Most margarine is also made using this process. Margarine

was first introduced as an inexpensive alternative to butter, but when the health benefits of unsaturated oils became evident, the marketing focus changed and they were heavily promoted as a *healthy* alternative to butter instead—only they haven't turned out to be all that healthy after all because most brands, especially stick margarines, contain trans fatty acids. The negative affects of trans fatty acids are primarily related to heart health. Trans fatty acids raise your bad cholesterol (LDL), raise your triglyceride level (another risk factor for heart disease), lower your good cholesterol (HDL) and may make some components in your blood stickier and more likely to form clots.

The FDA has recently passed new labeling regulations that will require trans fats to be listed on nutrition labels, but in the meantime, look at the ingredient list on the foods you buy. If it says "partially hydrogenated oil" or "vegetable shortening" it will contain some trans fats. Another large source of trans fat is fried food in restaurants, especially fast-food establishments. Use these foods sparingly if at all. If consumer demand diminishes, manufactures will be encouraged to use healthier alternatives.

At the other end of the continuum are omega-3 fatty acids. Interest in omega-3 fatty acids surged when it was learned that the Inuit peoples of Alaska and Greenland had very little heart disease, particularly atherosclerosis, despite the fact that they consumed large amounts of fat and cholesterol. This evidence was in direct contrast to what was the prevailing belief at the time—that diets high in fat increased your risk of heart disease. Investigation into this paradox revealed that their diets were high in fat, but they were also rich in omega-3 fatty acids, particularly EPA and DHA which were derived from the marine animals that made up a large part of their diets. These fatty acids improve heart health by improving the ratio of good cholesterol to bad cholesterol, making the blood less sticky and less likely to clot, reducing arrhythmias (erratic heart beats which can lead to sudden death), and reducing inflammation which is also an important factor in heart disease.

Continued research has shown that the beneficial effects of these fatty acids aren't just limited to the heart. Because they comprise a large part of the brain some advocates are raising the possibility that omega-3 deficiency could play a role in schizophrenia, attention deficit hyperactivity disorder, Alzheimer's disease, Parkinson's disease and autism. Studies have also shown it to be effective in reducing depression and the symptoms of multiple sclerosis. Because of its role in inflammation, it may be beneficial for people with autoimmune diseases such as arthritis, and it may reduce the symptoms of pre-menstrual syndrome—and the list goes on. More research is needed to fully understand the relationship of omega-3's to health and disease, but there is sufficient evidence right now to recommend that everyone should include fish or another good source of omega-3 fatty acids in their diet *at least* three times per week, but preferably every day.

Omega-3's are essential, meaning that you can't make them so you must eat them, but they aren't as easy to come by as they once were due to current manufacturing and agricultural processes. Because omega-3's easily oxidize and become rancid quickly, manufacturers partially hydrogenate them to improve the shelf life of their products, and farm raised animals and fish are fed grains high in omega-6 fatty acids instead of their natural diets which are high in omega-3's. For example, in their natural environment, wild salmon feed primarily on tiny shrimp-like crustaceans called krill, which contain a pink carotenoid called astaxanthin. Omega-3's are created by algae and other ocean plants which the krill consume and pass on to the salmon along with their lovely natural pink color. Farm raised salmon are separated from this natural food chain and are fed primarily grains such as corn which is high in omega -6 fatty acids and doesn't contain astaxanthin. As a result, farm raised salmon does not contain as much omega-3 as wild salmon does, and in order to make the flesh pink so that it will look the way consumers expect it to, farmers must add colorants to the feed. It may also contain more polychlorinated biphenyls (PCBs) which are potentially cancer causing chemicals, than wild salmon does.

It is possible to include omega-3 fatty acids in feed and produce a product which contains higher levels of these fats. Chickens which have been fed a vegetarian diet rich in omega-3 fatty acids produce eggs which are higher in omega-3 fatty acids. These eggs are already available in the marketplace and hopefully other foods with higher levels will be available soon. For right now the best sources of omega-3 fatty acids are fatty, cold water fish like mackerel, herring and salmon. Other, leaner fish like swordfish, flounder, cod and haddock contain less. Vegetarian sources are flaxseeds, walnuts and their oils. These oils should be kept in a dark, airtight container in the refrigerator to prevent oxidation. High quality fish oil supplements are also a good option.

Omega-3 fatty acids come in different chain lengths. The longer chain acids which are found in fish seem be more effective at improving health than the shorter chain ones found in vegetarian sources. The body can convert short chain acids into long ones, but it requires a larger amount of these fatty acids to obtain an equivalent amount of benefit. The ratio of omega-6 fatty acids to omega-3 also appears to be important. You should try to limit your intake of omega-6 fatty acids found in vegetable oils like corn, soy and safflower and use olive and canola oils which are high in omega-3 fatty acids instead.

So how much fat should you eat each day? There are many different guidelines that can be referenced. The FDA recommends that your total intake of fat should be less than 30 percent of calories and that saturated fat and trans fat should be less than 20g per day. In my experience most people find numbers and percentages difficult to put into practice, especially since individual needs can vary so much, so I suggest the following guidelines:

- Avoid trans fatty acids as much as possible. Don't order fried foods in restaurants and read package labels carefully.
- Reduce your intake of saturated fat. Use low fat or non-fat dairy products or substitute soy ones. Choose vegetable sources of proteins, fish, and poultry instead of red meat. If you eat red meat, purchase lean cuts, trim all visible fat away, and consume smaller portions. Remove the skin and visible fat from poultry as well.
- Limit your intake of non-nutritious "junk foods" high in fat like chips, baked goods and ice cream.
- Use monounsaturated oils like olive and canola freely and in place of polyunsaturated oils like corn and safflower, but don't overdo it because they are still high in calories. Remember moderation is the key.
- Enjoy high fat foods like nuts and avocado as part of a healthy diet, not in addition to one.
- Be sure to get some omega-3 fatty acids each day by consuming fish, flaxseeds, walnuts or their oils, or omega-3 enriched foods. High quality fish oil supplements are a viable alternative.

Another Reason to Avoid Fried Foods

Most commercially fried foods whether they come from a restaurant or a package are likely to be high in trans fats, but now there is a new concern. Cooking starchy foods like potatoes at high temperatures has recently been found to produce acrylamide, a chemical that may cause cancer and other health problems.

FAT SUBSTITUTES

The only substituting you need to do is good fats for bad fats and don't eat more than you need. Some fat substitutes interfere with your body's ability to absorb precious nutrients like the fat soluble vitamins A, D, E and K and can cause intestinal distress. Also, they don't help to stabilize blood sugar the way that natural fats can. Fat isn't an enemy of good health, used appropriately it is a valuable ally!

6

MICRONUTRIENTS: SMALL BUT MIGHTY

Vitamins are compounds that your body requires in very small amounts. They help to regulate vital body processes including the digestion, absorption and metabolism of other nutrients. Minerals are inorganic substances that the body uses both for building tissue and maintaining normal functions. If you follow the instructions for eating in this manual and you eat lots of fruits, vegetables, and whole grains, enough fish, poultry or soy, and use mainly monounsaturated fats for cooking and at the table, you will be getting most of the vitamins and minerals you need from your food, but taking a multiple vitamin and mineral supplement is still a good idea. Even if you are eating an organic, whole food diet, you don't eat all foods every day and there will be fluctuations in your daily intake. Your body stores some vitamins but not others, so taking a supplement ensures that you get enough of the basics each day.

Due to changes in agricultural practices and degradation of the soil, the nutrient content of some foods has diminished over the past half century. In conventional farming, the emphasis has been on improving appearance, storability and transportability, more so than on improving the nutritional value of fruits and vegetables. Most crops are bred to produce higher yields, to be resistant to disease, and to produce more visually attractive fruits and vegetables. As a result many fruits and vegetables don't contain as many vitamins and minerals as they once did. Many don't taste as good as they used to either. This is one of the many reasons why I recommend buying organic whenever you can. Organic farming practices result in better quality soil and more nutritious foods.

Supplements are an effective way to make up for shortcomings in the food supply or in your diet, but they should never be a substitute for healthy eating. Like fortification or enrichment, supplements only contain a few isolated nutrients, not the myriad of healthful compounds found in whole food. They can't make up for a poor diet or bad habits. They should be used as insurance only. Having insurance on your car doesn't mean that it's OK to drive carelessly or recklessly and taking supplements doesn't mean that it's OK to eat carelessly or recklessly.

You need enough vitamins and minerals to achieve optimal health but no one is certain exactly how much enough is. Most of the data we have regarding intake levels of vitamins and minerals is based on how much of these nutrients is necessary to prevent deficiency diseases such as scurvy with a cushion built in to account for normal growth and maintenance. Their role in the development of chronic diseases such as cancer and heart disease is still under investigation and not fully understood. However the most current findings suggest that getting more of these micronutrients than most people currently consume could be beneficial to long term health. The problem is that there isn't enough research available yet on many vitamins and minerals to know *how much* more. Until more information is available, moderation remains the best approach.

Vitamins and minerals don't work alone, they work in

conjunction with the foods you eat. When you get the micronutrients you need from your diet, everything remains in balance. A person who needs more food to maintain health would also need more vitamins and minerals to maintain health. By eating more food, they would get more vitamins and minerals—an efficient arrangement that works well for the body. When we use supplements to get extra vitamins and minerals we must take greater care because supplements are a more concentrated source of vitamins and minerals, and they are not being delivered in the natural packaging that your body is equipped to manage. Concentrated supplements can overwhelm your system's built in safeguards if you take too many or too high a dose. It's difficult to get too many vitamins and minerals from your diet, but it's not difficult at all to get too much from supplements. Taking more vitamins and minerals than you need can be just as unhealthy as not getting enough.

Taking high doses of water soluble vitamins means extra work for your liver to process them and your kidneys to dispose of them. If you are taking high dose supplements and your urine is very intense in color, you are taking too much. Fat soluble vitamins are stored in fat tissue and can reach toxic levels if you overdo it.

Taking excess minerals can also cause problems. Too much zinc for instance can impair your sense of taste and smell, cause your hair to fall out, suppress you immune system and raise your bad cholesterol while lowering your good cholesterol. It can also interfere with your body's ability to absorb copper. Most minerals require special vehicles to transport them from your digestive tract into your blood. Taking too much of one mineral may tie up a large number of these vehicles leaving too few to transport other minerals that require the same vehicle.

For instance, if you take too much calcium it can interfere with your body's ability to absorb iron.

For most healthy people a multivitamin and mineral supplement that provides 100% of the Daily Value is more than enough to insure adequacy. Remember you are taking this 100% *in addition* to what you are getting from your food, including enriched and fortified foods. Some servings of breakfast cereals contain as many vitamins and minerals as supplements do!

A healthy diet together with a multi-vitamin and mineral supplement will address most of your micronutrient needs, but there are a few vitamins and minerals that warrant special attention.

Antioxidants

Oxygen is a good thing to have in your body; without it you couldn't live very long. But oxygen also produces free radicals, tiny electrons that bombard your cells wreaking havoc wherever they go. Oxidative damage increases your risk of heart disease, cancer and some researchers believe it is the basis for most of the aging that occurs in your body. Antioxidants include Vitamins C, E, Beta carotene, the minerals selenium and zinc, and a host of phytochemicals such as lutein and lycopene. We know that in populations that eat the most fruits and vegetables (which are naturally high in these antioxidants,) the incidence of almost all chronic diseases is lower than in those populations that don't. We also know that each antioxidant has specific functions; no one antioxidant prevents all types of oxidative damage. What we *don't* know for certain yet is if isolating these antioxidants from nature's packaging and taking them as supplements will have the same effect. As I've mentioned before, nutrients don't work alone, they work in harmony with each other like a giant orchestra. We know that the symphony of nutrients found together in fruits and vegetables lowers your risk of disease and improves you health, but we don't know how much good any single instrument will do on its own. The best way to take advantage of antioxidants is to eat your fruits and vegetables!

Vitamin B$_{12}$

As you age your ability to absorb Vitamin B$_{12}$ may diminish and the absorption of this vitamin may also be impaired by the use of antacids, other medications and alcohol. A Vitamin B$_{12}$ deficiency can cause muscle weakness, tingling sensations in the arms and legs, confusion, memory loss, and can lead to other more serious health problems. A high intake of another B vitamin, Folate, which is now added to the food supply to prevent a type of birth defect, can mask this deficiency allowing damage to your nervous system to continue undetected. Vitamin B$_{12}$ is found in meat products so getting enough is also a concern for Vegans, people who eat no animal products whatsoever. A supplement is an easy way to make sure you are getting enough of this important vitamin. The current Recommended Daily Intake (RDI) is 6 mcg.

Folic Acid (Folate)

Folic acid is an important B vitamin. A deficiency of folate can lead to the development of neural tube defects, a type of birth defect that occurs during the first few weeks of pregnancy. It can also impair your body's ability to process homocysteine, an amino acid that can increase your risk of heart disease if your blood levels become elevated. You should be certain that you are getting the RDI of 400 mcg daily. Most multiple vitamin supplements contain this amount but read the label to be sure.

Vitamin C

Smokers break down Vitamin C faster than non-smokers do. Their need for Vitamin C may be as much as double that of someone who does not smoke. The current RDI for Vitamin C is 60 mg, but if you smoke heavily you will need much more, or better yet, quit smoking!

Vitamin D

Your body can make all the Vitamin D it needs if it is exposed to bright sunlight for about 15 minutes each day. For people who spend most of their time indoors due to weather, work, or disability, getting enough Vitamin D may be a problem. If you live in the Northern half of the United States where cold winters keep you indoors or covered up, if you work inside all day, or are confined to a nursing home, you are not likely to get enough exposure to sunlight to produce sufficient Vitamin D. The only good source is fortified dairy products, so if you don't consume dairy, make sure that your supplement contains 100% of the recommended amount which is 400 IU per day.

Vitamin E

Vitamin E is an antioxidant, and there is significant evidence that taking extra Vitamin E may be beneficial to your health. The current RDI is 30 IU, but a supplement of 400 IU per day may be helpful. Even though it is a fat soluble vitamin which the body can store, Vitamin E does not appear to be toxic at higher doses. However, it thins the blood and makes it less likely to clot, so if you are taking any medications for this purpose, check with your health care professional before including extra Vitamin E.

Calcium

Calcium is critical to overall good health, not just for building strong bones, but getting enough can be difficult. Dairy products are a good source but to get enough calcium from dairy products alone you would have to drink 3-4 glasses of milk each day, and dairy products are not a source of Vitamin K which is necessary for proper use of the calcium. Dark green leafy vegetables are a good source of both calcium and Vitamin K, but few people eat enough to get all they need. The recommended amount of calcium changes based on your age, but for most healthy adults an extra 1000 mg is plenty. Because fitting that much calcium into a multi-vitamin and mineral supplement would make it too large to swallow, you need to take a calcium supplement separately. Calcium is absorbed best when it is taken with food. If you are taking more than 500mg, spread your dose across more than one meal. Take one tablet with breakfast and another with dinner.

Iron

During their child bearing years women lose iron with each menstrual period. They also tend to eat less red meat than men and so are at higher risk for an iron deficiency which can leave them feeling tired, weak and can make concentration more difficult. A multivitamin and mineral supplement that includes the RDI of 18 mg of iron is appropriate for these women.

Men on the other hand, tend to eat more red meat and don't have a routine method for excreting excess iron so they *should not* take supplements that contain iron unless recommended by their health care professional. Studies have shown that an elevated level of iron can increase the risk for heart disease and that it might increase the amount of free radicals in your body. To lower iron levels, donate blood regularly. You may be able to save two lives at once.

Potassium

If you are taking diuretic medications which can cause you to lose potassium, or if you exercise for longer than ninety minutes at a time, you may need a little extra potassium. You can easily get what you need from a glass of orange juice, a bowl of spinach, a banana or a sports drink. Salt substitutes that contain potassium instead of sodium can help you increase your potassium intake and reduce your sodium intake at the same time.

Salt and Sodium

The average American diet contains anywhere from five to fifteen times the amount of sodium necessary to maintain good health, with most of the excess coming from processed foods. High levels of sodium intake are a concern because they may elevate blood pressure. Though not everyone seems to be sensitive to this affect, cutting back on sodium seems to be an effective way to reduce your risk of developing this silent killer. Ideally you should consume no more than 2400 mg (about 1 teaspoon of table salt) of sodium per day from all sources.

The best way to avoid excess sodium is to follow the recommendations in this manual for eating whole foods as close to the way nature created them as possible. There are no naturally occurring foods that are high enough in sodium to be a concern for good health. When you do use processed foods, be sure to read labels. The highest concentrations of sodium are found in foods that are prepared in brine like pickles and sauerkraut, smoked and cured meats and fish, snack foods, fast foods, canned and instant soups, tomato products, and condiments.

To help cut back on your sodium intake, replace salt in cooking with acids such as flavored vinegars or lemon juice. Garlic and herbs like basil, ginger and mint add lots of flavor too. Adding a little salt at the table instead of during cooking puts it on top of the food where you can readily taste it rather than in the food where you will need more to get the same effect. Many chefs swear by sea salt claiming that its larger crystals contain more minerals than regular salt which gives it more flavor.

BUYER BEWARE

There are thousands of different options in the marketplace when it comes to vitamin and mineral supplements. Nutritional supplements are not regulated by the FDA the way that medications are so there is no guarantee that what is on the label is what is in the bottle. When it comes to purchasing supplements the following guidelines may be helpful:

NATURAL VS. SYNTHETIC

With the exception of Vitamin E, there is no advantage to "natural" vitamins and minerals over synthetic ones except that they may not contain artificial colors which should be avoided whenever possible. Your body can't tell the difference if Vitamin C came from rose hips, oranges or a test tube. In fact, to get it from rose hips into that nice little white tablet, it had to be chemically extracted anyway. Fancy ingredients don't usually do much other than imply that a product is worth paying a higher price for. One exception is Vitamin E. Natural Vitamin E is better utilized by the body than synthetic Vitamin E, but the synthetic version will also work fine. You just need to take a little more of it to get the same effect.

WHAT'S IN THE BOTTLE?

Choose reputable brands. Large companies are usually careful to assure the quality of their products. Most store brands are fine and may be less expensive than those that are heavily advertised. If you want to be sure that you are getting what you think you are, check with an independent testing company such as consumerlab.com which provides independent test results to help consumers evaluate products. The CL Seal of Approval guarantees that a product has passed testing and any brand that carries the USP symbol has met the manufacturing standards of the United States Pharmacopeia; the same standards that are used for prescription drugs.

7

BUYING AND PREPARING HEALTHIER FOOD

A trip to the grocery store can be like finding your way through a maze. There are so many products to choose from, and the aisles are lined with goods and gimmicks positioned to entice you to buy what grocers and manufacturers want you to buy, not necessarily what you should buy. The aisles themselves are like mini prisons; once you enter at one end, it's difficult to turn around until you get all the way to the other end, which of course means that you are a captive audience to shelves and shelves of products strategically placed and temptingly advertised. The highest profit products that the grocer wants you to buy are placed at eye level or on special displays, while the products that you are most likely to buy without prompting line the lowest shelves. Cereals targeted at children are usually placed lower because that's where kids eyes are most likely to see them. Interestingly, "health foods" are either in a section of their own or on the highest shelves because consumers that want them are usually willing to search for them.

The best way to maneuver through the market is to spend as little time in the prison as possible and purchase most of your foods along the perimeter instead. That is where the fresh foods and most of the whole foods are located. Around the outer edges of the market is where you will find the produce section for fresh fruits and vegetables, the dairy cases, the meat and seafood departments and the bakery. Obviously there are many products that you will need from the main aisles, but shop for them from a list and read all labels carefully. A list helps you stay focused on what you want to buy and avoid impulsive purchases. Reading labels helps you to make the healthiest choices. A complete guide to understanding food labels is included in the next chapter. Once you become familiar with which foods meet your expectations or requirements, you won't have to read the labels as often.

Over time, you will come to know what products to buy and which to avoid. In order to keep your cold foods cold and prevent spoilage, you should always shop for refrigerated and frozen foods last.

FRESH, FROZEN OR CANNED?

Fresh food is best if it's *really* fresh. Once food is harvested, its nutritional value, quality and taste begin to deteriorate. We are fortunate to have year round access to fresh fruits and vegetables from all over the world, but items that have been in storage or transport for days or weeks before they reach your grocer's shelves, then sit in the drawer of your refrigerator for a few more days or weeks, don't really qualify as "fresh." Try to buy fruits and vegetables frequently rather than stocking up, and choose ones that are in season or produced locally. They are usually the freshest and also the least expensive. Farmer's markets are a great place to get fresh produce.

Fresh frozen fruits and vegetables are also an excellent choice and take a lot of the work out of preparing healthy meals. Cleaned and frozen right at the point of harvest, they will retain all of their nutritional value, color and taste. But be careful about using frozen prepared meals. They are processed much more and often contain sauces high in fat or sodium. Be sure to read the ingredient list and nutritional information on the label.

For seafood and meat products, a lack of freshness not only affects the taste and nutritive value, but the safety as well. If you don't have access to fresh caught seafood, Frozen At Sea (FAS) is the way to go. Many of today's fishing vessels are also processing plants. The catch is prepared, flash frozen, and vacuum sealed within minutes assuring a high quality, safe product. Many of the finest restaurants use FAS seafood products because the quality is better, there is less waste, and it's easy to store.

Canned products are OK in a pinch, but they are often processed at high temperatures which can destroy some of the nutrients. Most canned products also contain higher levels of salt or may have sugar added to them, so read labels carefully. Buy seafood packed in water rather than oil.

Buy dry goods in bulk when available and recycle your grocery bags or use reusable ones. However, never reuse plastic bags that have been used to wrap raw meat, poultry or seafood.

THE KEYS TO SUCCESSFUL SHOPPING

1. Make a list of what you need to buy and only buy what's on your list.
2. Never grocery shop when you are hungry.
3. Buy most of your foods from the perimeter and spend as little time as possible in the "prison."
4. Read the labels on everything until you become familiar with which products work for you.
5. Buy fresh if it's really fresh, or frozen is fine.
6. Buy fresh produce frequently so it is as fresh as possible.
7. Buy in season and locally grown if possible.
8. Use canned goods mainly as a back up for fresh or frozen, and check for additives, especially salt, sugar and oil.
9. Buy refrigerated and frozen foods last.
10. Buy in bulk and bring your own bags or recycle those supplied by your store.

HEALTHY FOOD PREPARATION

Starting with whole, fresh food is important, but so is how you prepare it. Boiling is fine for eggs, but boiling vegetables will cause them to lose many of their nutrients, so steaming or microwaving is a better choice. Either way, save the remaining liquid to use for soups and stock. It contains most of the nutrients that the vegetables lost and it will be more flavorful than starting with plain water. Sautéing, stir-frying, baking, broiling and roasting don't require the addition of much fat so they are far better choices than frying. Grilling can be healthy too, but fat dripping onto hot coals can form harmful chemicals that then rise with the smoke and are deposited on the food. To minimize this, use leaner cuts of meat so there is less fat to drip, or block the smoke with a sheet of foil. Slow cookers and microwaves offer convenient options for food preparation as long as you avoid recipes that call for lots of added fats or heavy sauces. You can also add flavor to food by marinating it, experimenting with seasonings, and cooking with wine, flavored vinegars and broths.

DON'T OVERCOOK YOUR FOOD!

Even when it comes to food preparation, *enough is better than more!* Overcooking destroys precious nutrients and can result in the formation of cancer causing compounds. We have known about the problems with overcooking meats for a long time, but a new concern in this area is the recent discovery that cooking carbohydrates at high temperatures leads to the formation of acrylamide. Acrylamide is known to negatively affect the nervous system and can cause cancer, so cook your carbohydrates, especially potatoes at the lowest possible temperature for the shortest period of time to reduce your exposure.

There is also some concern about using non-stick cookware at high temperatures. It appears that some of the compounds used in making the surfaces slick release harmful gases when the pans are heated too high. Instead of using non-stick cookware, use healthy fats likes olive and canola oil to keep your food from sticking.

UNDERSTANDING FOOD LABELS

Reading food labels is the best way to figure out what you are buying and how it fits into your overall plan for a healthy diet. Food labels are meant to be a source of information to help you make better decisions, but if you don't fully understand how they work, they can be misleading. One common mistake that people often make is not adjusting the information listed on the label to match how much food they actually eat. If the serving size used for the label is 2 ounces, but you eat 4 ounces, you have to multiply all of the nutrient amounts by two in order to get accurate information. If a serving size is 1 cup, but you only eat 1/2 cup, then you must divide the nutrient amounts in half. Though standardized for convenient product comparisons, the serving sizes listed on labels often differ from what people actually consume.

A second concern lies in understanding which terms and claims have legal meanings and which do not. "Low fat" means that a product has less than 3 grams of fat per serving, but "low carb" has no legal meaning; it doesn't guarantee anything with regards to how much carbohydrate the product contains. Imaginative names may imply that a product is healthier than it actually is.

Upcoming changes to the nutritional labels will make it easier to know how much trans fat you are getting, and there are new guidelines for what health claims can be included on the label, but the basic information included here will remain the same.

INGREDIENTS

Ingredients must be listed in descending order by weight. That means that whatever is at the beginning of the list is what there is the most of in the product, and what it contains the least of is listed last. The ingredient list doesn't give you absolute amounts, only relative ones. If the first ingredient is water and the second ingredient is fruit juice, you know that there is more water than fruit juice, but not how much more.

The ingredient list is most useful for identifying ingredients that you want to avoid such as artificial colors, flavors, preservatives, and other additives, and for managing food allergies. It is also valuable in confirming whether or not what the name of the product implies is what you are actually getting. In the carbohydrate chapter I used the example of bread products that use creative names which give you the impression that they are whole grain products when in actuality, they may only contain a very small amount of whole grain or none at all. This type of subtle deception isn't limited to grain products. It can be found on many products throughout the grocery store, so check your ingredient labels carefully to be sure you are buying what you think you are.

Note: If you have a concern about a product, most manufacturers offer toll-free numbers you can call to ask specific questions about a food product or ingredient.

THE NUTRITION FACTS

There are key elements to look for in the nutrition facts box. The serving size, the number of servings per container, the amount of calories and how many of those come from fat, the

Nutrition Facts

Serving Siz 1 cup (228g)
Serving Per Container 2

Amount Per Serving

Calories 260	Calories from Fat 120

	% Daily Value*
Total Fat 13g	20%
Saturated Fat 5g	25%
Trans Fat 2g	
Cholesterol 30mg	10%
Sodium 660mg	28%
Total Carbohydrate 31g	10%
Dietary Fiber 0g	0%
Sugars 5g	
Protein 5g	

Vitamin A 4%	•	Vitamin C 2%
Calcium 15%	•	Iron 4%

*Percent Daily Values are based on a 2,000 calorie diet, Your Daily Values may be higher or lower depemding on your calorie needs:

		Calories	2,000	2,500
Total Fat	Less than		65g	80g
Sat Fat	Less than		20g	25g
Cholesterol	Less than		300mg	300mg
Sodium	Less than		2,400mg	
2,400mg				
Total Carbohydrate			300g	375g
Dietary Fiber			25g	30g

Calories per gram:

Fat 9	•	Carbohydrate 4	•	Protein 4

amount of each nutrient, including fats, carbohydrates, protein and certain vitamins and minerals, the % Daily Values and Daily Values.

The serving size tells you how much of the product all of the other numbers are based on. If you eat more or less than this serving size, you must adjust the rest of the numbers to match. If you aren't sure how much you usually eat in grams, ounces or cups, you might find the number of servings per container easier to work with. For example, if you know that you are going to eat a whole bag of chips, but the servings per container are listed as 2½, then simply multiply the nutrient information by 2½. If a package says that it contains four 1/2 cup servings but you know that *your* family of four will eat two packages, then you also know that you have to double the rest of the information on the label. The serving size is important, but what really matters is how many of these servings you are going to eat.

The calories tell you how much energy the product will provide your body, and the number of calories from fat is helpful if you are trying to cut back on how much fat you eat. The sample label shows you that almost half the calories in this product are from fat.

The total amount of fat a serving contains is listed in grams, and that number is further broken down into saturated fat and *trans* fat. On the sample label, the product contains 13g of total fat, 5g of saturated fat and 3g of *trans* fat. That means that of the 13g of total fat, 7 grams—or more than half of the total fat—are the bad fats that you want to avoid. The remainder is made up of unsaturated fats, but there is no way to tell whether they are monounsaturated or polyunsaturated without reading the ingredient list to see what type of oils were used to make the product. The amounts of cholesterol and sodium are listed next, followed by the carbohydrates. Like the fats, the carbohydrates are broken down further to let you know how much of the carbohydrate the product contains is dietary fiber and how much of it is sugars. The more fiber a product contains the better, but it's best to avoid products that are too high in sugar. Protein is listed next, also in grams.

For each of these nutrients a % Daily Value is included. Based on a 2000 calorie per day diet, the Daily Values are provided to assist you in relating the nutrient amounts to the rest of your diet. They help you decide if the 13g of fat found in our sample product is a lot or a little. If you normally eat 2000 calories per day, according to national recommendations you should get no more than 65g of fat in your diet. The sample product contains 20% of your total fat for the day, but 25% of your saturated fat allotment. Again, if you want accurate information, you have to do some math. If you normally eat only 1500 calories per day, your total fat intake should not exceed 50g, so this product actually contains 26% of your total fat for the day.

Vitamins A, C, calcium and iron are the only micronutrients required on the food label. Manufacturers may list others if they so choose. Below the vitamins and minerals, the total Daily Values are included for your information as is the number of calories found in fat, carbohydrate and protein.

LABEL DICTIONARY

By law, certain terms used on food labels have specific meanings, but unfortunately, others do not. Low fat means that the product contains 3 grams of fat or less per serving, but low carb doesn't have a legal definition, it is a marketing term only. The core terms which do have legal definitions are:

- **Free:** This term means that a product contains no amount of, or only trivial or "physiologically inconsequential" amounts of, one or more of these components: fat, saturated fat, cholesterol, sodium, sugars, and calories. For example, "calorie-free" means fewer than 5 calories per serving, and "sugar-free" and "fat-free" both mean less than 0.5 g per serving. Synonyms for "free" include "without," "no" and "zero." A synonym for fat-free milk is "skim".
- **Low:** This term can be used on foods that can be eaten frequently without exceeding dietary guidelines for one or more of these components: fat, saturated fat, cholesterol, sodium, and calories. Thus, descriptors are defined as follows:
  — **low-fat:** 3 g or less per serving
  — **low-saturated fat:** 1 g or less per serving
  — **low-sodium:** 140 mg or less per serving
  — **very low sodium:** 35 mg or less per serving
  — **low-cholesterol:** 20 mg or less and 2 g or less of saturated fat per serving
  — **low-calorie:** 40 calories or less per serving.

Synonyms for low include "little," "few," "low source of," and "contains a small amount of."

- **Lean and extra lean:** These terms can be used to describe the fat content of meat, poultry, seafood, and game meats.

— **lean:** less than 10 g fat, 4.5 g or less saturated fat, and less than 95 mg cholesterol per serving and per 100 g.

— **extra lean:** less than 5 g fat, less than 2 g saturated fat, and less than 95 mg cholesterol per serving and per 100 g.

• **High:** This term can be used if the food contains 20 percent or more of the Daily Value for a particular nutrient in a serving.

• **Good source:** This term means that one serving of a food contains 10 to 19 percent of the Daily Value for a particular nutrient.

• **Reduced:** This term means that a nutritionally altered product contains at least 25 percent less of a nutrient or of calories than the regular, or reference, product. However, a reduced claim can't be made on a product if its reference food already meets the requirement for a "low" claim.

• **Less:** This term means that a food, whether altered or not, contains 25 percent less of a nutrient or of calories than the reference food. For example, pretzels that have 25 percent less fat than potato chips could carry a "less" claim. "Fewer" is an acceptable synonym.

• **Light:** This descriptor can mean two things:

—First, that a nutritionally altered product contains one-third fewer calories or half the fat of the reference food. If the food derives 50 percent or more of its calories from fat, the reduction must be 50 percent of the fat.

—Second, that the sodium content of a low-calorie, low-fat food has been reduced by 50 percent. In addition, "light in sodium" may be used on food in which the sodium content has been reduced by at least 50 percent.

The term "light" still can be used to describe such properties as texture and color, as long as the label explains the intent—for example, "light brown sugar" and "light and fluffy."

- **More:** This term means that a serving of food, whether altered or not, contains a nutrient that is at least 10 percent of the Daily Value more than the reference food. The 10 percent of Daily Value also applies to "fortified," "enriched" and "added" "extra and plus" claims, but in those cases, the food must be altered.

Alternative spelling of these descriptive terms and their synonyms is allowed—for example, "hi" and "lo"—as long as the alternatives are not misleading.

- **Healthy:** A "healthy" food must be low in fat and saturated fat and contain limited amounts of cholesterol and sodium. In addition, if it's a single-item food, it must provide at least 10 percent of one or more of vitamins A or C, iron, calcium, protein, or fiber. Exempt from this "10-percent" rule are certain raw, canned and frozen fruits and vegetables and certain cereal-grain products. These foods can be labeled "healthy," if they do not contain ingredients that change the nutritional profile, and, in the case of enriched grain products, conform to standards of identity, which call for certain required ingredients. If it's a meal-type product, such as frozen entrees and multi-course frozen dinners, it must provide 10 percent of two or three of these vitamins or minerals or of protein or fiber, in addition to meeting the other criteria. The sodium content cannot exceed 360 mg per serving for individual foods and 480 mg per serving for meal-type products.

OTHER DEFINITIONS

The regulations also address other claims. Among them:

- **Percent fat free:** A product bearing this claim must be a low-fat or a fat-free product. In addition, the claim must accurately reflect the amount of fat present in 100 g of the food. Thus, if a food contains 2.5 g fat per 50 g, the claim must be "95 percent fat free."

- **Implied:** These types of claims are prohibited when they wrongfully imply that a food contains or does not contain a meaningful level of a nutrient. For example, a product claiming to be made with an ingredient known to be a source of fiber (such as "made with oat bran") is not allowed unless the product contains enough of that ingredient (for example, oat bran) to meet the definition for "good source" of fiber. As another example, a claim that a product contains "no tropical oils" is allowed—but only on foods that are "low" in saturated fat because consumers have come to equate tropical oils with high saturated fat.

- **Meals and main dishes:** Claims that a meal or main dish is "free" of a nutrient, such as sodium or cholesterol, must meet the same requirements as those for individual foods. Other claims can be used under special circumstances. For example, "low-calorie" means the meal or main dish contains 120 calories or less per 100 g. "Low-sodium" means the food has 140 mg or less per 100 g. "Low-cholesterol" means the food contains 20 mg cholesterol or less per 100 g and no more than 2 g saturated fat. "Light" means the meal or main dish is low-fat or low-calorie.

- **Standardized foods:** Any nutrient content claim, such as "reduced fat," "low calorie," and "light," may be used in conjunction with a standardized term if the new product has been specifically formulated to meet FDA's criteria for that claim, if the product is not nutritionally inferior to the traditional standardized food, and the new product complies with certain compositional requirements set by FDA. A new product bearing a claim also must have performance characteristics similar to the referenced traditional standardized food. If the product doesn't, and the differences materially limit the product's use, its label must state the differences (for example, not recommended for baking) to inform consumers.

'Fresh'

An FDA regulation defines the term "fresh" when it is used to suggest that a food is raw or unprocessed. In this context, "fresh" can be used only on a food that is raw, has never been frozen or heated, and contains no preservatives. (Irradiation at low levels is allowed.) "Fresh frozen," "frozen fresh," and "freshly frozen" can be used for foods that are quickly frozen while still fresh. Blanching (brief scalding before freezing to prevent nutrient breakdown) is allowed.

Other uses of the term "fresh," such as in "fresh milk" or "freshly baked bread," are not affected.

Health Claims

As of September 2003, in order to include a health claim on a label or package, a product will have to go through a new health claims review process that is designed to encourage marketers of foods and dietary supplements to make accurate claims about the health benefits of their products and to discourage the use of false or misleading claims. The new system will grade claims based on the quality and strength of the scientific evidence supporting them. If a claim receives an "A," its use will be allowed without further qualification. A grade of "B," "C," or "D" will require a disclaimer.

8

A Roadmap for Restaurant Dining

M ost Americans eat a minimum of 25% of their meals away from home. For some people that number may be as high as 65% to 70%. An occasional break from eating healthfully to indulge in dining at a favorite restaurant might not have serious long term consequences, but when restaurant food becomes a staple in your diet, the choices you make when eating out become very important.

An average restaurant meal contains between 1000 and 2000 calories and 50 to 100 grams of fat. A deep fried whole onion with sauce at one popular restaurant chain contains 1438 calories and 114 grams of fat and it's only considered an appetizer! If you followed it with one of their jumbo burgers and fries, which contains another 1476 calories and 76 grams of fat, (mostly saturated and trans) you will have consumed 50% more calories than most people need for an entire day, and 190 grams of fat at one meal. That's three times the recommended amount of fat you should eat per day, and most of it is the bad stuff you want to avoid.

Portion size and fat content are just two of the many obstacles to eating nutritiously when you are away from home. Limited menu options, omnipresent advertising, and dessert tray temptations are also common challenges you will face. Most of these obstacles can be overcome by a little planning and learning how to choose wisely. The major challenges of dining out are:

- Not eating more than you need to
- Avoiding too much of the wrong kind of fat
- Avoiding too much salt
- Finding nutrient dense foods
- Getting enough fiber
- Avoiding temptation

Not Eating More Than You Need To

As you learned in the beginning of the EAT section, going too long between meals can cause a drop in blood sugar that makes you feel ravenous and can easily lead to overeating. If it has been more than three hours since your last meal, have a light snack before you head to the restaurant. Doing so will help you to have greater control over how much you eat. But counting on self control alone to stop eating when there is a whole plate of delicious food sitting in front of you is a recipe for disaster, especially if your are over-hungry. If you are like most people, if it's there, you will eat it, even if you don't intend to. You may get distracted by an interesting conversation or the company of others, and the next thing you know, your plate is empty. Or you might put your fork down and say you are finished, but then fall prey to what I fondly refer to as "Oh, just one more bite" syndrome. You know that you are full and don't really need to eat any more, but it tastes so good that you're just going to have one more little taste, only you keep on tasting away until you finish it all or the waiter removes the plate.

The best way to avoid overeating is to not have more food than you want, or need to eat, sitting in front of you. Have anything you don't want to eat like bread, rolls, or chips removed from the table, and when you order your food, order less. Many appetizers are just the right size to be a meal, and lots of restaurants offer half size or lunch portions on request. You can also order one meal and share it with a dining companion. If it's not quite enough for two, adding an extra salad is an easy way to get more nutrients without a lot more calories. If you do order a whole meal for yourself, ask your server to bring you a take out container when he brings the meal. Before you even take the first bite, remove the portion of your food that you don't want to eat right then and place it in the container. You would probably have to be extremely hungry to open the container and start eating from it while still in the restaurant so this can be an effective strategy for reducing your serving size.

If you are dining at a buffet, extra caution is necessary because it's easy to get carried away. Use a salad size plate instead of a dinner plate, and make additional trips through the food line if you need too. Keep in mind that an all-you-can-eat sign is an invitation to eat what you care to, not a personal challenge to see how much you can eat.

To help you feel full faster and increase your fluid intake at the same time, remember to drink a large glass of water before you begin to eat.

Avoiding Too Much Fat—Especially the Wrong Kind of Fat

Stay away from fried foods as much as you can. They will not only be high in calories and fat, but most likely they will be high in trans fat—the worst fat on the healthy fat continuum. If you are ordering a starchy fried food like french fries, you also have to be concerned about acrylamide formation. Having foods that are grilled, broiled, baked or steamed is a better way to go.

Fried foods aren't the only sources of fat on the menu. Salad dressings, cream soups, gravies, sauces, cheeses, croissants and desserts are all going to be high in fat, most of it saturated fat or trans fat. You are the customer and you are in charge so don't be afraid to ask for your food to be prepared the way you want it. Request substitutions like fruit instead of fries, and let your server know that you want your vegetables without butter and your sauce, gravy, cheese, or dressings either left off or on the side. To reduce the amount of salad dressing you use, try dipping your fork into the dressing before picking up a bite of your salad. You will have a little bit of dressing on every bite, but use very little dressing overall. Better yet, make your own dressing using olive oil and vinegar and ask for olive oil instead of butter for your bread. It will replace the saturated and trans fats with monounsaturated fat and a little omega-3.

WORDS OF CAUTION

The following words are all nice ways of saying "Loaded with fat!"

buttered	creamed	au gratin	béarnaise
double crusted	crispy	au lait	beurre blanc
hollandaise	crunchy	au fromage	encroute
escalloped	gravy	a la mode	pan fried

prime (prime meat is more tender because it contains more fat)

Avoiding Too Much Salt

Avoid foods that have salt you can see on them like chips or margaritas. Ask your server to have your food prepared without salt, and to bring all sauces, gravies and dressings on the side. Many are very high is salt. Taste your food before reaching for the salt shaker and only apply what you really need to make your food taste better. Use condiments like ketchup sparingly; they too are often high in salt or sodium.

Finding Nutrient Dense Foods

The same foods that are nutrient dense at home like fruits, vegetables, whole grains, lean meats, poultry, seafood, and dairy products are nutrient dense in restaurants, as long as they haven't been smothered in fat during preparation. If you are dining at a restaurant that has a very limited menu, ask if they have any substitutions available. Even a restaurant that doesn't serve salad can at least offer you lettuce and tomato slices which they might otherwise use as a garnish. Double up on the nutrient dense foods that are available and cut back on the ones that aren't. You can always balance one meal of lower nutritional value with one of higher nutritional value elsewhere in the day.

Getting Enough Fiber

Go for the whole grains whenever possible and ask for a double serving of vegetables or an extra salad instead of potatoes, white rice, or pasta. Have fresh fruit like berries or cantaloupe for dessert.

Avoiding Temptation

Recent research has shown that certain parts of the brain light up when exposed to dessert foods like vanilla ice cream. It hasn't been determined yet whether this is a conditioned response because you have always been taught that dessert is special, or because of some physiological reason, but it leaves little doubt that the best way to avoid temptation is to do just that—avoid it. Ask your server to remove dessert menus and advertising that may be on your table and not to bring by a dessert tray at the end of the meal. If you are dining with others who want dessert or you would like some, limit the amount you eat by sharing. If you want a treat and it's not too late in the day for caffeine to be a problem, order a dessert coffee like a cappuccino. Even with a little whipped cream on top it's a better choice that most other dessert alternatives except for fruit. If a meal just isn't a meal without something sweet at the end, carry a small treat with you like a lollipop. A little extra sugar won't be a big problem after a meal, and a small treat will contain less calories and less fat than anything available on the menu.

Try to dine at restaurants that offer healthier options. Restaurant menus are required to meet the same standards for accuracy as food labels are, so if an item carries a name like "low fat," it should be just that, low in fat. Many restaurants also use symbols to show which items on their menus meet the recommendations of a particular organization such as the American Heart Association. When available, use these labels and symbols to make healthier selections.

II. MOVE

9

GET YOUR BODY IN GEAR AND MOVE!

The importance of activity and exercise in remaining healthy simply can't be overstated. The human body was meant to move, not to sit at a desk, in front of a TV, or behind the wheel of a car. Almost any ailment that you can name from lower back pain to cancer will have some relationship directly or indirectly to a lack of movement.

Evolution is a slow process. It can take millions of years for significant change to take place in the body, but the world we live in has been changing at incredible speed. The human body, its components and systems evolved to equip man with the ability to acquire the necessities of life—food, shelter, and clothing—and to assure his survival in a harsh environment. In a primitive world this meant hunting and gathering, building or adapting a place to live, and responding to frequent physical threats. Just staying alive required a lot of physical work. Life remained physically demanding even through the early stages of the industrial revolution, but with the arrival of each labor saving device created to make our lives easier or more productive, our need for physical activity has diminished. It is entirely possible in today's world to meet all of your needs for survival without even standing up! You can order whatever you need on-line, by phone or mail and have it delivered right to your door.

Modern life is designed to discourage movement rather than encourage it. We have moving sidewalks and moving stairs, automatic dishwashers, carwashes, and a remote control for everything. But the human body has not had enough time to adapt to all of this convenience and we are paying for it with our health.

When my parents were children, their families grew much of their own food. In order to eat, the land had to be worked and the animals tended. When I was a child, making dinner meant a daily visit to the local markets, which were all within walking distance. We would head to the butcher for meat, to the produce market for fruits and vegetables, to the bakery for bread, and to the grocer for anything else we needed. Driving to the supermarket was only an occasional event to stock up on items that weren't readily available or too expensive locally, like laundry detergent. In order to eat, you didn't have to work, you only had to walk. Now, my family and I live in a typical suburban community and we drive to the supermarket for most of what we buy. We don't have to do much work or walking in order to eat. We just eat. Lack of movement combined with processed convenience type foods is an important contributor to our very modern day epidemic of obesity.

If you want to be healthy, you have to move your body. It's that's simple. Moving your body improves the strength and efficiency of your heart, your lungs, and helps keep your muscles firm and strong. It helps build stronger bones, gives you more energy and burns fat. Moving on the outside keeps things moving on the inside too. It improves the circulation of blood and helps prevent constipation. The more you move, the better you will feel physically and mentally. People who move more are less affected by stress, experience less depression and anxiety, and less premenstrual syndrome than those who move less. They also sleep better, have fewer illnesses and injuries, and they live longer.

If you want to feel great and look your best, you have to get moving. Movement includes both activity and exercise. **Activity** includes everything that you do other than sleeping or sitting at rest. If you are preparing dinner or mowing the lawn, that's activity. Chasing after your children is activity and so is shopping for a large screen or plasma TV. No matter what you are doing, if it involves standing and moving it counts as activity and there are lots of easy ways to increase your total activity level throughout the day.

Exercise is any activity that develops or maintains physical fitness. It requires more effort than simple activity, but it doesn't have to mean joining a gym or a baseball team. Anything that challenges your body enough to increase your heart rate by 50%, builds muscle, or increases your flexibility counts as exercise. Classic forms of exercise like jogging, swimming or weight training are great but so are ballroom dancing, playing hopscotch with your kids, and a round of golf. Physical labor that involves lifting, carrying, or moving your body against gravity like climbing a ladder is also exercise.

Both activity and exercise contribute to your overall health and can reduce your risk of illness and disease. Being active is far better than being sedentary and adding regular exercise improves your health even further. It is important to note that the health benefits of exercise are transient. When you stop working out, it doesn't take long to lose the gains you've made. Getting fit and remaining fit is a life long process.

Regardless of your age, activity and exercise will help you to feel and look your best and improve the quality of your health. The earlier you start, the better, but it's never too late. Studies have shown that adults in their 80's can still build muscle and improve their cardiovascular condition with regular exercise. People who remain physically active feel better, look better and have more energy to live life than people who don't. So get moving!

10

ACTIVITY

Increasing your activity level poses few if any risks so you can get started right away, but if you have been sedentary, are over the age of 45, or have any medical conditions, it's important to see your health care provider before you embark on an exercise program.

There are many things that you can do throughout the day to increase your activity level. For instance, while you are waiting for an appointment, standing instead of sitting in a chair keeps your heart rate up a little higher and burns a few more calories. When you get tired of standing and sit down, you can keep your body moving by tapping your foot or squeezing and releasing the muscles in your buttocks. Both require muscle contractions, and utilize energy. If done frequently and consistently these little increases in activity can lead to firmer muscles and burn hundreds of extra calories each day. The following strategies don't require much effort, but every little bit helps and the cumulative impact of these small but valuable changes in the way you approach life can be significant.

Doing The Daily Dozen—Twelve Simple Ways to Increase Your Activity Level

1. Stand Instead of Sit Whenever You Can

Standing requires more energy and effort than sitting does and it increases your heart rate.

2. Walk Instead of Ride

Whenever you can use your legs instead of your wheels you will be contributing to your activity level. Park further from your destination and walk the rest of the way. Take the stairs instead of the elevator.

3. Be Your Own Motor

If you do use wheels, power them with your muscles instead of gas. Instead of driving, ride a bike or rollerblade. It will be better for your health and will help reduce air pollution.

4. Reduce Your Use of Convenience Appliances

Pretend it's the good old days and get up to change the channel or adjust the volume on your TV. Stand and hand chop your vegetables instead of using a food processor. Use a push lawn mower instead of a riding one.

5. Look Into Their Eyes

Make it a personal rule to always get up and go speak to someone instead of using the phone, intercom, or calling across the room whenever you can. Doing so will get your body moving *and* improve the quality of your communications.

6. Do It to Music

Whatever you are doing, doing it to music will make you move more. When doing routine chores, listening to upbeat music will make you move faster and with more force. You might even find yourself throwing in a few dance steps along the way. Music makes most activities seem to go by faster, so you are also likely to engage in them longer.

7. Fidget

Forget what your mother said. According to a study done at the Mayo Clinic, when it comes to burning calories and keeping your activity level up, there is no advantage to sitting still. If you must sit, tap your toes, bounce your knees or drum your fingers. Just be considerate and try not to annoy others.

8. Stand Up Straight

OK, this time, *do* listen to your mother. Maintaining good posture, changing your body position often, and stretching frequently all add to your total activity level.

9. Do Your Chores

Routine tasks that require movement such as washing the car and folding laundry are actually good for you.

10. Flex Your Muscles

Contracting and relaxing your muscles counts as activity even if no one can tell you are doing it. Squeezing the muscles of your buttocks while you sit in a chair increases your activity level and can improve your muscle tone at the same time. Squeezing a tennis ball in your hand can help you relieve stress while you are stuck in traffic. Pulling your belly button towards your spine and holding it during a red light or a television commercial will help to flatten your tummy. Sucking in your gut is a good thing to do.

11. Find a Hobby You Enjoy

Any hobby that requires you to move is a good choice. For example, gardening involves working with the earth, carrying water and fertilizer, and pulling weeds, all of which require movement.

12. Get a Dog

Dogs need to be trained, walked, fed and groomed, all of which require activity from you. Besides they are great companions who can make activity more pleasurable.

11

EXERCISE

The goal of exercise is to develop or maintain your strength, flexibility, muscle endurance, and cardiovascular/respiratory fitness. Strength training builds muscle and speeds up your metabolism, while flexibility improves your balance and helps reduce your risk of injury. Muscle endurance helps prevent your muscles from becoming fatigued, and cardiovascular conditioning increases the strength and efficiency of your heart and lungs. It also improves circulation. Weight bearing exercises lead to an increase in bone mass and help to prevent bone loss and fractures associated with osteoporosis.

As you can see different types of exercises contribute to your overall fitness in different ways and to differing degrees. Weight training builds muscles and improves your strength, but doesn't do much for your flexibility. A dance class keeps you flexible and improves your cardiovascular health, but doesn't increase your muscle strength very much. A good fitness plan incorporates a variety of exercises that together improve all four aspects of fitness and result in total body conditioning.

How much exercise do you need to stay healthy?

There are three factors which need to be considered when determining how much exercise you need:

> **Frequency:** How often you exercise
> **Duration:** How long you exercise
> **Intensity:** How hard you exercise

Your individual health and fitness goals will influence how you blend these elements and how much of each you need. If your goal is to simply improve your health, you will need to do some form of exercise such as walking a total of 30 minutes per day, most days of the week. However if you wish to achieve physical fitness, it will take a bigger commitment on your part. In order to maintain cardiovascular fitness as well as healthy body composition—meaning enough muscle tissue and not too much body fat—your fitness plan should include:

Aerobic Exercise:

- 3–5 Times per week
- Continuously for 20 to 60 minutes
- At a moderate to strong level of exertion. Try to remain in your target heart rate zone which is 60–90% of your maximum heart rate (See instructions for determining your maximum heart rate)

Resistance Training:

- 2–3 Times per week
- At least one set of 8–12 exercises for each major muscle group, multiple sets if time allows
- With sufficient intensity to enhance strength. To build

muscle tissue, use greater resistance and perform less repetitions or sets. To increase muscle endurance, use less resistance and do more repetitions.

Flexibility Training:
• A minimum of 2 -3 times per week
• For 10 -30 minutes
• Without straining

If you have a medical condition careful monitoring of your heart rate may be necessary, but an easy way to estimate if you are in your target heart zone is to try and speak. You should be able to talk normally, but not be able to sing. If you are breathing so hard that you can't speak, slow down, you're working too hard. If you have no trouble singing the National Anthem, you probably aren't working hard enough. The more fit you become the more efficient your heart will be resulting in a lower resting heart rate.

ESTIMATING YOUR TARGET HEART RATE

To measure your resting heart rate per minute, place your first two fingers (not your thumb) on a pulse point under your chin or on the inside of your wrist and count how many beats occur in 30 seconds, then multiply this number by 2. To determine your maximum heart rate, subtract your age from 220. To determine your target heart zone, multiply this number by 0.6 and 0.9 or use the table below. These heart rates are only an estimate and can vary depending on your age, sex and level of fitness but they are a useful guide for beginning an exercise program.

Target Heart Rates

Age	Maximum heart rate per minute	55%	90%
20	200	120	180
25	195	117	176
30	190	114	171
35	185	111	167
40	180	108	162
45	175	105	158
50	170	102	153
55	165	99	149
60	160	96	144
65	155	93	140
70	150	90	135
75	145	87	131

FIRST THINGS FIRST—SAFETY

Before you begin a new exercise program remember to check with your health care provider, especially if you are over 45, have a medical condition or are taking any medications. Once you have the all clear, the following guidelines will help to keep you safe and injury free.

Always Warm Up Before You Exercise

A five to ten minute gradual increase in activity helps to warm the muscles and make them more flexible and less likely to tear. It also gives your heart rate a chance to rise slowly.

Stretch

Don't try to stretch muscles during your warm up or when they are cold. Wait until they are warm, then take a few minutes to stretch them before beginning your exercise.

Use Proper Equipment Including Safety Gear

The right equipment can make the difference between a pleasant exercise experience and a disaster. Make sure that all of your equipment meets current standards and fits properly. When exercising at night, be sure to wear reflective clothing and carry or wear a light. And don't forget sunglasses, sunscreen and bug repellent if you are exercising outdoors.

Don't Wear Headphones on Busy Streets and Always Walk or Run Facing Traffic

Contact with moving vehicles may be hazardous to your health. You need to be able to hear and see what is going on around you to protect yourself from danger on the road.

Don't Forget Your Feet

Your shoes should fit well and be designed for the exercise that you are participating in. Running shoes are specifically designed to support forward motion and cushioned to minimize impact. Court and aerobic shoes provide extra support for lateral motion. Athletic shoes need to be replaced often, even if they don't look worn. Many exercise related injuries are due to poor fitting or inappropriate footwear.

Wear the Right Clothing

The right clothing like the right shoes should fit your body and your sport. For cold weather activity layering provides extra warmth. As your body or the weather warms, layers can be removed to accommodate the change. In both warm weather and cold, loose fitting clothing that "wicks" water away from the body is helpful.

Learn from a Pro

Before you take on a new sport be sure to get the proper instructions. In every sport there are factors that can affect your safety and no instruction or poor instruction can lead to injury.

Set Realistic Goals

Getting fit takes time. As we get older our bodies manufacture less growth hormone and may respond to exercise more slowly. But even if you aren't seeing rapid results, exercise is still beneficial to your health.

Let Your Motto be "No Pain, No Strain."

When starting a new exercise program it isn't uncommon to experience some discomfort, but exercise shouldn't hurt. You don't have to "Go for the burn" to get a good workout. Listen to your body and let it be your guide. Take your time and increase your exercise gradually.

Frequency, Duration, Intensity—Increase Only Once at a Time

Don't try to go from a 30 minute program 3 times per week to an hour long program 5 times per week. Build your workouts up slowly. Trying to do too much too fast can lead to injury and increased soreness.

Pay Attention to Your Form

Proper form and body alignment assure a safe workout and maximum benefit from your exercise.

Maintain Proper Hydration

Make sure you take in enough fluids. Drink before, during, and after exercise to remain fully hydrated. It will improve your performance and lessen the chance of your experiencing a heat related illness. Hydration is just as important in cold weather as it is in warm weather. If you exercise strenuously for more than 60–90 minutes, or in hot humid conditions, a sports drink that replaces electrolytes and carbohydrates may be useful, otherwise plain water is fine.

Cool Down

Never just stop at the end of your workout; it can cause a sudden drop in blood pressure. Instead gradually reduce the intensity of your exercise and allow your breathing to return to normal.

AEROBIC EXERCISE

Aerobic means "with air." Aerobic exercises are those activities that require a larger than normal volume of oxygen to be available to your muscles. In order to meet this increased oxygen demand the number of red blood cells (the ones that carry oxygen) increases and your heart muscle becomes stronger, allowing it to pump more blood with each beat. This improved efficiency makes fewer beats necessary so your heart rate decreases and your resting blood pressure is more likely to remain normal. The muscles that support the action of your lungs also become stronger making your breathing more efficient as well.

Regular aerobic exercise leads to improved cardiovascular endurance and better circulation throughout the body. It also reduces your risk of heart disease by raising blood levels of HDL, the "good" cholesterol, and lowering blood levels of LDL, the "bad" cholesterol. Insulin and glucose are handled more effectively which reduces your risk of diabetes and metabolic syndrome—also known risk factors for heart disease.

But aerobic exercise isn't just good for your heart. Improved circulation benefits your whole body. Every organ, tissue and cell is better able to obtain the nutrients they need and dispose of their wastes. Increased oxygen flow to the brain improves cognitive function and memory, and causes the release of endorphins. Endorphins are your body's natural "feel good" hormones. They reduce anxiety, depression, and pain, and leave you feeling relaxed and happy. They are the chemicals responsible for what is known as "The runner's high," a feeling of euphoria experienced by some people after sustained periods of exercise. Aerobic exercise reduces the level of stress hormones in the blood. Since stress hormones impair immune function and disrupt sleep, regular exercisers are less likely to get sick and more likely to get a good night's sleep.

Perhaps one of the most important benefits of aerobic

exercise is its role in helping you to maintain a healthy weight. Obesity increases your chances of having high blood pressure, high cholesterol, a heart attack or a stroke. It increases your risk of developing cancer of the breast or colon, diabetes and all of its complications, arthritis and gall stones. It can even make you snore or become infertile.

As was discussed in the EAT section of this manual, weight management depends on maintaining a balance between how many calories you take in and how many your body spends. Aerobic exercise helps tip the energy balance in favor of controlling or losing weight by helping to burn off extra calories. A 150 pound person can burn anywhere from 100 to 300 extra calories by doing 30 minutes of aerobic exercise. That's enough to offset a slice of cake or four chocolate chip cookies. But the good news doesn't stop there. Because aerobic exercise requires sustained activity, it encourages the burning of *stored* fat.

Normally, your muscles use a combination of glucose (sugar), fatty acids (fat) and a little protein for fuel. Your body can only store small amounts of sugar but even the leanest person has energy to spare stored as fat. Because the need for fuel in aerobic exercise remains high for more than a couple of minutes, your body realizes that it will run out of glucose if it doesn't change the fuel mixture. That would have very serious consequences, especially for your brain and nervous system which depend primarily on glucose for fuel. (Athletes know this condition as "hitting the wall.") In order to avoid depleting glucose stores, the body shifts to burning a higher percentage of fat, most of which must come from storage sites around the body. You can't control where the body will draw fat from—there's no such thing as "spot reducing," but the total amount of fat in your body will be reduced.

Your body will continue to burn more fat even after you stop exercising because your metabolic rate will remain elevated for some time. Studies have shown that the more intensely you exercise, the longer your metabolic rate remains higher, but it varies from person to person. Thanks to the reduction in stress hormones and the increase in endorphins that aerobic exercise brings about, you are less likely to engage in stress related eating or to crave fatty foods which might lead to regaining the fat that you have lost. Aerobic exercise is an important tool in effective weight management.

To be considered "aerobic," an exercise must be sustained for at least 20–30 minutes and raise your heart rate to at least 55% of your maximum heart rate. Any activity that uses the major muscle groups can meet these requirements. High impact aerobics can put a lot of strain on your bones and joints so consider low impact activities if you have problems with your knees, hips or back. If jogging isn't your thing, ride a bike or take an aerobics class. You can go for a swim, ski cross-country or downhill, or challenge a friend to a game of tennis or racquetball. Choose an activity or several that you like. Variety helps keep you from getting bored and since no single exercise works every muscle group, cross training is a good way to achieve total conditioning.

Swimming is an excellent exercise that can be enjoyed by everyone, even those with physical limitations such as arthritis or obesity. Because there is no impact involved and the body is supported by water, swimming does not stress your bones or joints, yet it works almost all of the major muscle groups, improves muscle strength and endurance, and is aerobic. Heart rate does not usually increase as much with swimming as with other aerobic activities so it doesn't burn fat as efficiently, but this does not reduce it's effectiveness in overall body conditioning.

THE KEYS TO AEROBIC EXERCISE

- Always warm up before you begin and cool down when you are done.
- Always stretch after you are warm and at the conclusion of your workout.
- You must continue your activity for at least 20–30 minutes. The longer you continue to exercise, the more fat that you will burn.
- Make sure that you are properly hydrated. Drink before, during and after exercise.
- Don't overdo it. It's better to build up slowly than to risk injury. If you overdo it, you many not be able to work out again for several days.

RESISTANCE TRAINING

When regularly challenged with resistance, your muscles and the supporting tissues that work with them like tendons and ligaments, adapt by growing stronger. So do the bones that lie beneath them. These structures together with your organs make up what is called your lean body mass. Lean body mass is very metabolically active. It burns lots of fuel, produces heat, and allows you to do work. It is the engine that runs your body. Without regular resistance training your muscles and everything related to them begin to break down and weaken as you age. As the amount of lean body mass declines, so does your metabolism, and a slower metabolism means that you must either eat less or you will gain weight. Many of the conditions we attribute to aging such as muscle weakness and "middle age spread" are really not caused by aging, but by a lack of exercise and a reduction in lean body mass.

Body fat is not very metabolically active. It more or less just hangs around taking up space, and it takes up more space per pound than lean body mass does. A person who is leaner will be smaller and have a much more toned, fit appearance than a person of equal height and weight who is less lean. Stronger muscles also improve your posture helping you to look taller and thinner and reducing back pain.

A strong body performs better under all conditions than does a weak one. Whether you are doing routine daily tasks or responding to a physical challenge, with a stronger body everything will seem easier.

Muscle strength is measured as the maximum force that a muscle can produce. Muscle endurance is how long the muscle can work before it becomes fatigued. Together they determine how hard and how long you are able to perform any given task, including exercise. To increase the strength and endurance of your muscles, you must use resistance training. Resistance training involves the overloading of a muscle group. This overloading causes microscopic tears to form in the individual muscle fibers. The muscle heals itself by adding extra protein to fill in the tears which increases the size and strength of the muscle. How large and strong muscles become is affected by how hard you train and your genetic makeup. Without the use of dangerous growth enhancing hormones and steroids, women cannot build the same type of large muscle structures as men, and not all men have the genetic potential to become Mr. Universe.

The greater the amount of resistance you use in training, the larger and stronger your muscles will become. To continue building new muscle, you should use enough resistance to exhaust your muscle with 8–12 repetitions of the exercise, and the amount of resistance must be progressive. That means that as your workout becomes easier for you, you need to add more resistance if you want to continue building new muscle tissue. To increase muscle endurance you need to use less resistance and do more repetitions.

The resistance can come from free weights such as barbells and dumbbells, weight training machines like those found in most gyms and health clubs, portable resistance devises such as hand and ankle weights and elastic tubes, or the weight of your own body. Yoga, some Pilates exercises and plain old fashioned push ups all use the body as resistance.

Traditional weight training is not an aerobic activity. Your heart rate may increase considerably and quickly while you are lifting, but does not remain elevated when you rest between sets. Circuit training is a modified form of resistance training that usually involves the use of weight training machines. You use a moderate amount of weight, complete several repetitions, and move quickly from one machine to the next without resting in between. This type of workout works well for those with limited time to devote to an exercise routine.

Isometric exercises offer another way to fit resistance training into your life. They can be done anywhere, anytime and require no equipment. An isometric exercise involves using an immovable object such as a wall for resistance or contracting opposing muscles against each other. Standing in a doorway and pushing against both sides of the frame or clasping your hands together tightly while trying to pull them apart are examples of isometrics. They are not nearly as effective as traditional resistance methods, but any exercise is better than none. Isometrics are a great way to get in a little resistance training when you are confined to a location for extended periods of time such as flying in a plane or while at the office.

THE KEYS TO RESISTANCE TRAINING

- **Seek professional guidance.** It is very important to use correct form and the proper amount of weight for resistance training. A certified personal trainer can design a program that's right for you.
- **Work with a partner.** It's more fun to have the company and encouragement of a companion when training, but when strength training with free weights it is also a matter of safety. You should always have a person spotting you who can help you to control your weights in the event that your muscles give way.
- **Always warm up before you begin training.** Don't train cold muscles. They will injure easily.
- **Don't hold your breath.** It raises your blood pressure significantly and can be dangerous. Always exhale on exertion and inhale on relaxation.
- **Work each muscle group to exhaustion.** The point of resistance training is to overload the muscles either by using a heavy weight or using a moderate weight and doing more repetitions.
- **Rest between sets.** Muscles need a chance to recover.
- **Don't work the same muscle group two days in a row.** Give your muscles at least two days between workouts. If you strength train every day, alternate between muscle groups. Train you upper body one day and your lower body the next.
- **Stretch.** Always stretch your muscles at the end of your workout.

FLEXIBILITY TRAINING

There is a belief in Chinese medicine that the longer a person's hamstring muscles, the longer they will live, so I spend a lot of time reaching for my toes. Improved flexibility may or may not extend your life, but it will extend your range of motion and reduce the likelihood of your sustaining an injury. Regular stretching relieves stiffness and helps prevent muscle cramps and low back pain. It improves your balance making you less likely to fall and it's a great way to reduce the effects of stress.

Stretching can be as simple as stretching your hands over your head and reaching for the sky or as complex as an advanced yoga posture. Either way, it is an important part of your total exercise program.

THE KEYS TO FLEXIBILITY TRAINING

- **Always stretch *after* your muscles are warm** and after you finish your workout.
- **Hold your stretch** for 20–30 seconds. You should build up to this length of time gradually.
- **STOP if you feel pain.** You might experience some discomfort when you first begin stretching, but it shouldn't be painful. Eventually, it will feel great!
- **Don't bounce!** Reach as far as you can, then inhale. As you exhale try to reach a little further. Bouncing can cause you to overstretch or injure your muscles.
- **Be patient.** The older you are and the longer it has been since you last stretched, the longer it will take for you to attain your flexibility goals, but don't despair. With regular practice you *will* get there.

FINDING TIME FOR FITNESS

For many people the biggest challenge of exercising is trying to fit it into their daily lives. The more demands there are on your time, the more difficult it may be, but it isn't impossible, especially if it becomes important enough to you. The problem for most people is that they consider exercise a luxury that gets done *after* all of the other important tasks of the day, rather than recognizing it for the necessity that it actually is and making it a priority in their lives.

No matter how busy you may be you probably wouldn't even think of not showering or brushing your teeth before you go to work, even if it meant being late. Why? Because looking clean, smelling fresh, and being socially acceptable is more important to you than most other things, and because you have accepted your daily hygiene practices as a non-negotiable given. They *will* get done. When you decide that exercise is just as important, it too *will* get done.

Here are a few tips to get you started:

- Schedule exercise into your day just as if it were an important meeting or appointment, *and treat it like it is one!*
- Commit to a partner. Sometimes it's easier to do something when you know someone else is counting on you. Having a partner that you agree to exercise with on a regular schedule may give you the extra push you need when it's difficult to get going.
- Combine exercise with other activities. March in place while you cook dinner, or conduct a business meeting on the golf course.
- Make exercise convenient. Plan activities that you can do easily and close to home or work. Keep exercise equipment

readily available so that if you have a few extra minutes you can use them for fitting fitness in. I travel with an exercise tube and use isometrics at my desk.

- Start your day a little earlier. Just a few minutes of exercise in the morning can improve your whole day.
- Break up your workout into small manageable bits. Take a walk break instead of a coffee break. Ten minutes in the morning, afternoon and evening equals the necessary 30 minutes a day
- Turn off the TV. Unwinding at the end of the day with a brisk walk will do more to relax you than watching TV. If you must turn on the TV, put in an exercise video.
- Play with your kids. A few minutes of one-on-one basketball or jumping rope is great exercise and sets a positive example for your child.
- Choose leisure activities that involve exercise like hiking or mountain biking. See the world instead of a movie.
- Avoid an "All or nothing attitude." A small or partial work-out is always better than no work out at all.

Don't wait until you have a health crisis, or an emotional one (like having to fit into a special dress for your upcoming high school reunion!) to make exercise a priority. Do it now.

III. RELAX

12

PUT THE BRAKES ON STRESS

Excess stress drains your energy, clouds your brain, destroys your health and robs you of joy. The ancient Greeks were well aware of stress and referred to it as disharmony or a lack of balance in the body. Without the benefits of modern medical technology they still understood that it was a contributor to disease. Somehow that understanding, like numerous other ancient treasures was lost for many years, and the importance of stress as a credible cause of physical illness was minimized. Instead it was viewed primarily as a mental or psychological problem. Gratefully, its relationship to physical health has been rediscovered and the research is conclusive: stress makes you sick. It can even kill you.

Not all stress is bad for you. Positive stress can be a powerful motivator and can inspire you to be more efficient—some people do their best work under pressure. It can also help condition you to be able to respond better in difficult situations. However when the amount of stress you are exposed to becomes too great, or you are unable to cope effectively with a particular type of stress, it becomes *dis*tress and *dis*tress can have a profound and negative affect on your health.

The stress response is a milder version of the powerful "fight or flight" response; an instinctive, carefully orchestrated series of biological and physiological events designed to help you survive in an emergency. In order to appreciate the power and value of the "fight or flight" response, imagine yourself back in prehistoric times just stepping out of your cave to greet the morning sun. You look up towards the sky and there, perched high above you on a rocky ledge is a very large cave lion that's looking at you and thinking "Breakfast!" Since he knows that you are there, only two choices remain: do battle with the beast or escape to a safer location. Either way, your body will respond by instantly flooding your system with stimulating hormones such as adrenaline and cortisol, along with extra fuel to help improve your performance and your chances of survival.

Your heart rate and blood pressure will increase, and so will the clotting ability of your blood. If you are injured, rapid clotting reduces the risk of your bleeding to death. Your liver will dump fat and sugar into your blood to provide additional fuel for your muscles and organs, and your respiration will increase to provide more oxygen. Since digesting what's in your stomach offers no immediate advantage, your GI tract will shut down allowing more blood and energy to be diverted to other parts of the body where they can be put to better use. Even the activity of your immune system will be temporarily suppressed. These are all wonderful things that are beneficial in a true emergency and they certainly helped primeval man to stay alive, but the "fight or flight" response is meant for dealing with serious threats which are infrequent and temporary. When this heightened state of readiness becomes a constant part of everyday life due to chronic stress, it's a whole different issue.

High blood pressure and blood that's more likely to clot may be a good thing if you are about to wrestle with a cave lion, but if they are ever present as a result of chronic stress, they are simply setting you up to have a heart attack. Impaired digestion can lead to everything from heart burn to irritable bowel disease and malnutrition. Chronic stress increases your need for extra nutrients, while at the same time making it more difficult to acquire them. Temporarily suppressing your immune system to help you escape a burning building or an attacker is fine, but long term suppression can make you much more susceptible to infection. Chronic stress has been estimated to contribute to 80% of all illnesses, including cancer. It can also impair your memory, lower your sex drive, and cause you to gain weight. But it doesn't have to be this way. There are lots of things you can do to reduce the amount of stress in your life and minimize the negative effects of the stress you can't eliminate. The most important thing to remember about stress is:

The only person who can manage the stress in your life is <u>YOU!</u>

Most of the circumstances and conditions of your life are a result of the choices you make. It's much easier to lay the blame for everything negative in your life on someone or something else besides you, but this sets you up to become an eternal victim and leaves you powerless to create change. Looking at your life honestly and accepting whatever responsibility in a given situation belongs to you empowers you to improve that situation. If you say "Look what he or she did to me" there is nothing you can do to make things better because you have no power to change another person. None of us do. We may think we can changes others, but that is an illusion. Change always comes from within. On the other hand, if you say "Look what I *allowed* that person to do to me," you *can* change things. You can *choose* not to allow them to do that to you again or you can *choose* not to allow it to affect you in the same way.

I once had a boss who was a typical "type A" personality. Everything in life was a crisis for him. He was a micro-manager and a control freak whose every decision was motivated by fear of failure. Working for him was incredibly difficult and yes, stressful. I used to find myself constantly complaining to friends and co-workers about the way he treated me and the things he did to me until one day, someone asked me why I tolerated his awful behavior and why I let him get to me so much.

At first I came up with lots of good reasons, like "I need this job," "Because he's in charge," "Because I want a promotion and if he doesn't give me good evaluations I won't get one." They all *sounded* like good reasons but the more I thought about it, the more I realized that they weren't good reasons at all. I was a valuable employee who did my job well, and being yelled at or getting upset by someone else's overreactions wasn't part of my job description. The only reason he was able to make me feel badly was because I was allowing him to.

It was an amazing revelation! From that moment on I practiced detaching my emotions from his. If he was upset about something, I acknowledged that he was upset, but I didn't get upset along with him. I *chose* not to. When he raised his voice, I turned down my hearing. Eventually, I took it one step further and when he raised his voice, I very politely pointed out to him that he was *shouting* at me and that I didn't hear him any better when he shouted than when he spoke more softly—and that was a revelation for him. He was so caught up in his own emotions that he hadn't even realized that he was shouting. Things

improved a bit, but old habits die hard so I took a firmer stand.
I politely told him that his shouting was unacceptable and if he
couldn't talk to me in a civil tone that I would have to quit. I
was very nervous confronting him and afraid that it might cost
me my job, but I knew that I wasn't willing to work under those
conditions any more anyway, it was just having too negative an
impact on the quality of my life. He didn't fire me and things
did get better, but not better enough, so I chose to find another
job. More importantly, I learned a valuable lesson:

No one can make you feel anything unless you allow them to.

Once I accepted the fact that I couldn't control his actions,
but neither could he control my re-actions, I no longer felt powerless in the situation. If the only reason that he was able to
upset me was because I allowed him to, I just wouldn't allow
him to any more. He could say or do whatever he wanted to,
but how I reacted to his words and actions was up to me. Just
knowing that made the situation less stressful.

I also used to get very stressed sitting in traffic. I felt like it
was a waste of time and I hate being late. When I was stuck in
traffic I could actually feel the muscles in my neck tighten, and
I would often arrive at my destination with a stress headache. I
was always blaming being late or not getting things done on "the
traffic" as if there was nothing I could do about it. Of course it
was the traffic's fault! It certainly wasn't my fault! Or was it?

I couldn't do anything about the traffic itself, but I could have
done things to lessen its impact on my life. I knew how heavy
the traffic was at certain times of day and in certain locations

and I also knew that getting stuck occasionally was inevitable, but I never did anything with that knowledge. Instead I continued to drive the same places at the same time and blame my problems on something "out there," the traffic, rather than accepting my share of the responsibility. However, once I did accept my fair share of the responsibility, I was empowered to do something about it; to improve the situation.

Now, I *choose* to listen to the traffic reports in order to avoid delays whenever I can. I *choose* to leave earlier to allow time for the unexpected, and I choose to keep books-on-tape and a voice activated tape recorder in my car so that if I am stuck in traffic, I can use the time effectively. I get some of my best ideas when my car is sitting still on a highway! The traffic is still the traffic, but now I have some control over how it affects me and that makes dealing with traffic much less stressful. This has taught me a second valuable lesson:

> ### *If you choose to believe that the causes of your stress are beyond your control then you deny yourself the opportunity to do anything about them.*

Feeling powerless to change a negative situation is very stressful. Knowing you have the power to change something and taking action to achieve that change empowers you to reduce the stress in your life.

REDUCING THE EFFECTS OF STRESS ON YOUR HEALTH

Consume a Nutritious Diet

Stress increases your need for nutrients while at the same time making them more difficult to acquire because it impairs digestion. The more malnourished you become, the more severely stress will impact both your body and your mind. Try to consume nutrient dense foods and follow the instructions in the EAT section to make sure that you are providing your body with everything it needs. The following nutrients are of special importance when you are under stress:

- **B vitamins:** Due to an increase in energy metabolism, these vitamins can be used up very quickly, and they are especially important in the functioning of the nervous system.
- **Antioxidants:** Beta carotene, vitamins C & E, and the minerals selenium and zinc. Stress promotes the formation of free radicals which can damage your body and speed up the aging process. Antioxidants help to prevent or reduce this damage. Other antioxidants include Coenzyme Q10, green tea, Pycnogenol (pine bark extract) and grape seed extract.
- **Calcium and Magnesium:** During the stress response the body is less able to store these minerals and they can become depleted.
- **Avoid excess caffeine:** Caffeine is a stimulant which can cause you to feel more agitated and stressed if you consume too much. Try taking a breathing break instead of a coffee break to help you relax or substitute a calming herbal tea such as chamomile.

Get Enough Sleep

When you are well rested you are much better prepared to cope with life and manage stress. When you are tired, everything seems more difficult and you are less able to deal with the challenges of life effectively, both mentally and physically. This can easily lead to more stress which can in turn make it more difficult to sleep. It is important to do everything you can to break this negative cycle.

Exercise

Physical activity gives your body a chance to respond to the "fight or flight"/stress response as it was intended to—by moving. In a true emergency, the influx of hormones and the physiological changes caused by the "fight or flight" response would be followed by a burst of activity; a fight or a flight. That burst of activity would exhaust the effects of the stress hormones, burn through the excess fuel in your system, and cause the release of *anti*-stress hormones called endorphins. Endorphins trigger the relaxation response and reverse the actions of the stress response leaving you feeling calm and peaceful. They also stimulate the pleasure centers in the brain leading to a feeling of joy or even euphoria. When no activity follows the stress response, the stress hormones remain in the system unabated, wreaking havoc all over the body, and much of the excess fuel ends up stored as fat. Exercise prevents this from happening while strengthening the body to better withstand the effects of stress overall.

13

Living a Less Stressful Life

Prevention is always preferable and usually more powerful than cure. Rather than trying to manage the stress in your life, it makes sense to prevent as much of it as you can in the first place, then manage what's left. The suggestions that follow are all helpful ways to lower you total stress load. Since we are all unique individuals, some of these suggestions may apply to you and the circumstances of your life more than others, but take the time to review them all because just as your mind and body are intricately interconnected and dependent on each other, so are the sources of your stress. For example, you may be a great time manager, but if you have too much stuff to take care of, make too many commitments, and take on responsibilities that don't belong to you, your time management skills won't lower your stress level. In fact, they may be allowing you to increase it by taking on more than you should.

Maybe time isn't an issue for you but dealing with frustration is. If you are surrounded by people who drive you crazy, or you are always angry at the world for one thing or another, you might find yourself tempted to live in the past wishing for the good old days, or in the future, putting your happiness on hold until "when." "I will be happy 'when' I get a new job, 'when' I lose weight, 'when' I win the lottery—'when' whatever." Living anywhere but in the moment is very stressful.

After reviewing all of the stress reduction techniques, choose the ones that are best suited to your needs, but always begin with identifying and prioritizing the sources of stress in your life. Knowing where you are going is required to get there, and knowing how to get there gets you there faster.

IDENTIFY AND PRIORITIZE THE SOURCES OF STRESS IN YOUR LIFE

Awareness is crucial to making effective changes. Without taking the time to clearly identify what the sources of stress in your life are, you could invest lots of time and energy making changes that will only provide a minimum of relief. To ensure that you get the maximum return on your investment and make changes that will make a substantial difference in your total stress level, follow these steps.

1. **Make a list** of the things that create stress in your life. As new thoughts come to mind, add them to your list.
2. **Prioritize your list.** Rank each item in descending order of *how much* and *how often* it contributes to your daily stress load.
3. **Select only one or two** of your major stressors to work on at a time. Trying to fix everything at once will only create more stress.
4. **Decide** what changes you can make that would improve the situation.
5. **Set specific goals.** For example, "I will listen to traffic reports and leave for work no later than 6:30 AM each day." Goals must be specific, realistic, and measurable.
6. **TAKE ACTION!** Thinking and planning are great, but you have to actually do something for change to occur.

7. **Remember** that managing stress is a process, not an event. The sources and types of stress in your life constantly change.

8. **Re-evaluate** your list on a regular basis. When one goal has been accomplished, set a new one.

LEARN TO MANAGE YOUR TIME

Time is a precious commodity. Everyone seems to need more of it, but unlike money, it can't be borrowed, saved for a rainy day, or charged to an account. Therefore you should make every effort to spend it wisely. Time is also the Great Equalizer because everyone regardless of age, sex, wealth, or power gets the same 1440 minutes each day. Feeling that you have too much to do and not enough time to do it can make you feel pressured and increase your stress level. Realizing that you have all the time there is, and adjusting your life to accommodate that limitation can help you to spend your time effectively and reduce your stress level.

Have a Plan and a Schedule for Each Day

A plan says what you are going to do. A schedule says when you are going to do it.

Prioritize Your Tasks

If you can't get everything done, it's better to choose the things that will get done and the things that won't rather than leaving that to chance.

Most Things Take Longer Than You Think

Planning unscheduled time into your day will allow space for the unexpected.

Start With the End in Mind

If you have to be somewhere at 8:00 PM, begin there and working backwards, deduct appropriate amounts of time for each task or activity that must take place before you go. This will ensure that you have enough time to prepare for your appointment and will help you to determine how much time you have available for other things.

Example: In order to arrive at 8:00 PM

- 30 minutes for driving
- 10 minutes to stop for gas
- 40 minutes for dinner
- 30 minutes to dress
- 10 minutes to pick up clothes at cleaners

= Begin to get ready at 6:00 PM

Get Organized

Create a place for everything and put everything in its place. Looking for things wastes time and increases both stress and frustration.

Anticipate Problems

Have an extra set of keys for everything, all of your work backed up on a computer disk and a plan for when things go wrong.

Learn to Delegate

You are not the manager of the universe and you don't have to do everything yourself.

Distinguish Personal Responsibility from the Responsibilities of Others and Learn to Say "No."

People who are efficient, effective, and dependable are often overburdened. Everyone counts on them for assistance because they know that whatever they need done, it will be done right, on time, and handled well. If you happen to be one of these people, it is important that you know where to set the limits for demands other people place on your life. Saying "No" isn't selfish. It is both responsible and generous. When you take on more than your fair share of responsibilities it takes a toll on the quality of your life and your health. When your life or your health becomes compromised, you have less to offer others.

Be as careful about giving away your time and your energy as you are about giving away your money. If you are a generous person, you probably donate money to help others from time to time or regularly. But you probably don't give so much of your money away that you don't have enough left to eat with or to pay your own bills. You are willing to be helpful but not at the expense of compromising your own safety or security. You need to apply the same standards to giving away your time and energy because they are far more precious than your money. The next time someone asks you to do something for them:

- Don't confuse guilt and manipulation with true responsibility.
- Remember that just because you can do something doesn't mean you *should* or *have to.*
- Be kind, generous, and supportive of others, but not at the expense of your own well being. If you don't take care of yourself, you won't have as much to offer others.

SIMPLIFY YOUR LIFE

It's easy to make things more complicated than they really are and to fill your life with "stuff" that you don't need but that you are still responsible for. Everything you possess and everything you commit to requires effort on your part to maintain. It's important to evaluate the objects and routines in your life and determine if they are really worth the stress they create. Just because you have always done something a certain way doesn't mean that it is the best way to do it or even that it needs to be done at all. Also be careful not to allow "stuff" to take over your life. If you have to work harder to earn more money to buy "stuff," then spend more of your precious time taking care of your "stuff," and worrying about your "stuff," you might soon find that you don't have enough time left to *enjoy* your "stuff," so what is the point in even having the "stuff?"

The simpler your life is, the less stress it will contain, so get rid of things that you don't need, don't enjoy, or that don't add value to your life.

LIVE IN THE PRESENT

What is in the past is just that, in the past, and beyond your reach. You can't change it, you can only learn from it, and appreciate it for what it was. Feeling powerless is very stressful and thinking about what "could" have been or "should" have been focuses your attention on things that you are powerless to change. There are no "do-overs" in life. It is far better to remain in the present where you *do* have power and you *can* make choices that affect change than to spend your time in the past where you can't.

Reliving fond memories is great fun and can be very relaxing, but remaining stuck in the past or constantly longing for that which no longer is also makes you feel powerless. No matter how hard you try or what you do, you *cannot* be younger again or re-create the wonderful past experiences of your life. Continually wishing you could will only increase your stress and interfere with your ability to fully appreciate the experiences open to you in this, the present moment.

Young children are wonderful at remaining in the present and keeping their bodies and minds in the same place at the same time. If they are playing with a friend, they play. If they are watching a favorite television show, they watch. Their bodies aren't playing or watching while their minds are off doing ten other things. Instead they are giving all of their attention to what is happening right now. We can learn a lot about living less stressful lives by watching children. They don't waste their lives or spend time fretting about what happened yesterday or worrying about what will happen tomorrow, they just live and enjoy being alive.

As adults we have responsibilities and obligations that children don't, but while these do give us things to be concerned about, they do not justify useless worrying. Understanding the difference between a concern and a worry is important. A *concern* is something that you can do something about, that you can affect in some way. A *worry* is something that you have no power to affect.

Being concerned about something allows you the opportunity to adjust your plans or your schedule to accommodate what lies ahead. Taking action to address a concern is productive and makes you feel more in control. For example, if you are *concerned* about the possibility of rain, you can allow extra time for driving and bring an umbrella or a rain coat with you wherever you go. Having prepared for the prospect of rain, you can forget about it and get on with your day.

Continuing to focus attention on whether or not it *will* rain is *worrying* because there is nothing you can do to affect it. The weather is beyond your control. If it's going to rain, it's going to rain whether you worrry about it or not. Continuing to worry about something that you cannot do anything about is unproductive. It is a waste of your time and energy that serves no purpose other than to increase your stress level.

The "fight or flight"/ stress response was meant to allow you to respond effectively to an emergency when one *actually exists.* Constantly triggering this response and remaining in a heightened state of readiness by worrying about an emergency that only *might* occur damages your health, depletes your body's resources, and simply wears your body out.

Whenever you find yourself feeling anxious about something, stop and ask yourself, "Is this a concern or a worry?" If it's a concern, then take action to address it. Do whatever is necessary so that you can stop thinking about it and then move on to other things. If it's a worry, acknowledge that there really is nothing you *can* do about it and let it go. To do anything else other than let it go would be a stressful waste of time and energy.

Don't Compare Yourself to Others

There will always be others who are more in some way than you are, and there will always be others who are less. Even for an Olympic gold medalist, his or her reign at the top is only temporary. Focusing on others can be very stressful, especially since you can't do anything about them. The only person you can change is yourself, so focus on doing your best and being all you can be and let others be concerned with themselves.

KEEP AN OPEN MIND

Things aren't always what they seem and you won't always be right, especially when you are trying to interpret the words or actions of others, and *how* you interpret those words or actions can have a tremendous impact on your stress level.

Most of us have experienced some occasion when we realized that something was not as we thought it was. We became upset about something only to find our emotions doing a quick about face when we discovered the truth. It's easy to judge the actions of others and to respond to them with strong emotions when they inconvenience or annoy you in some way, or if you suspect that they carry a negative intention. But it is healthier to recognize that there may be a reason you aren't aware of, or something that you don't fully understand that causes someone to behave in a certain way or causes a given circumstance to occur. Try to give people the benefit of the doubt, accept them for who they are, and have patience and compassion in dealing with them. It's much less stressful than getting angry.

GIVE PEOPLE A BREAK

No one is perfect and we all make mistakes, including you. Instead of getting angry at the blunders of others, try to give them a break and hopefully someone will do the same when it is your turn to do something foolish. If everyone did this, we would all have the pleasure of living in a kinder, friendlier, and less stress filled world. To err is human and some people are just more human than others.

I have a personal policy that entitles everyone, including myself, to one free pass for doing or saying something really stupid each day. It may sound silly, but it definitely lowers my stress level.

One day I was on my way to give a stress management presentation in front of a large audience. My flight had been delayed, my rental car wasn't ready when I finally landed, and despite all of my planning, scheduling, and leaving of extra time, I was still in jeopardy of being late. So instead of stopping for my usual healthful lunch, I went through the drive-thru at a fast food restaurant and grabbed a burrito. I knew I wouldn't have time to eat when I arrived, so I did something else I normally don't do, (and highly recommend that no one ever do!), I tried to eat while I was driving. Big mistake. *Huge* mistake.

Because I was in a hurry, I was driving in the far left, fast lane of a three lane road when all of a sudden a guy in the far right lane decides to make a *left hand turn!* Without even looking, he cuts across three lanes of traffic and right in front of me. Needless to say, I slammed on the breaks and squeezed the daylights out of my nice, juicy burrito. I narrowly avoided having a traffic accident, but the entire front of my suit was covered in refried beans and bright red hot sauce. In that instant I had two choices, I could either get very upset, roll down my window and start yelling at the driver for doing something so dumb, or I could simply say to myself "OK, there goes *your* free pass for the day!" Either way I was still going to have burrito filling all over me and I wasn't going to have enough time to do anything about it before my presentation. I always carry extra hose, extra contact lenses, and other emergency supplies with me when I speak, but I don't travel with an extra suit in my briefcase.

Getting upset wouldn't have changed my situation, but it would have changed my stress level and affected my performance on stage. It's hard to inspire others to be calm if you are upset. So instead of making matters worse by getting angry, I took a few deep breaths and continued down the road to meet my audience.

I got a few strange looks when I arrived and since there was no point in trying to ignore my appearance, I opened the program by telling the story of what had happened. I was able to use it as an example of what not to do— like eating and driving at the same time, and of how even great planning and scheduling offer no guarantees in life so you had best be able to accept the unexpected. It gave me an opportunity to demonstrate by example that controlling your reactions is not only possible, but that it can prevent the mistakes of others from ruining your day. Rather than being put off by my appearance, the audience found the whole situation amusing. It instantly broke the ice, made me more human and easy to relate to, and demonstrated that I *try* to practice what I preach which gave me greater credibility.

I gave the distracted driver a break and the audience gave me one in return. The simple act of choosing not to get angry turned what otherwise might have been an extremely stressful situation into a very positive experience instead.

MONITOR YOUR THOUGHTS

Thought precedes action and attitude is everything. These are not clichés, but valuable advice. If you fill your brain with negative thoughts, it will lead to negative feelings, words, and poor choices; all of which create stress. Positive thoughts, words and actions decrease stress. When you find your brain focusing on negatives, make a conscious choice to replace those negatives with something positive instead. When you hear the voice in your head saying things like "I can't do this," immediately replace that negative message with a more encouraging one, "I *can* do this," or "*How* can I make this work?"

When you find yourself thinking about bad things that *might* happen, unless there is something you can do to prevent them from happening, refocus you thoughts on something good happening instead. The more you practice doing this, the easier it will become and the calmer you will feel.

Be Flexible

A rigid tree branch breaks in the wind while a flexible one which can bend survives the storm. Palm trees thrive in warmer climates not only because of the weather conditions but also because they are able to survive hurricane force winds. I am always amazed at how dramatically mighty palms bend and sway in a storm. Some may be lost and others may lose their leaves, but when the storm subsides, most are there to live another day.

It is the same with people. Standing your ground and having to have things your way creates stress, especially in situations where you don't have control. If something is important enough or necessary enough, it may be worth the stress of insisting upon, but very often it is not. Choose your battles carefully. Remaining flexible and able to alter your expectations or adapt to change will reduce the amount of stress your body is subjected to.

Avoid Excess Noise

Noise pollution isn't just an annoyance, it's a health issue. It makes sense that chronic exposure to excessive noise can impair your hearing, but studies have shown that it also affects children's ability to learn, increases blood pressure, heart rate, respiration, muscle tension, and the presence of stress hormones in the blood. Some people may be able to adapt to noise on the conscious level by "tuning it out," but learning to ignore noise does not eliminate its physical affects. When test subjects felt they were not bothered by noise, or were no longer aware of it, their bodies still reacted to it.

Noise has psychological affects as well. People who are exposed to noise during their sleep often wake up feeling irritable and needing more rest.

Addressing noise pollution is a serious concern in the work place and some large cities like New York are taking action to improve noise levels on a community level. Reducing the noise in your personal environment is up to you.

- Fabric draperies, upholstered furniture and carpet absorb sound.
- Insulation in walls and ceilings can reduce noise within the home.
- Purchase appliances designed for quiet operation.
- Before moving to a new location, evaluate its noise level at various times of day. You should be able to hear someone speaking in a normal voice without difficulty when you are twenty-five feet apart from each other.
- Wear earplugs or sound proofing muffs when using loud equipment and avoid using that equipment late at night or early in the morning when it may disturb others.

Spending time in quiet, peaceful environments is an important step in reducing your total stress load.

LIMIT YOUR EXPOSURE TO TOXIC PEOPLE

Some people are a joy to be around. Being in their company or just speaking with them on the phone makes you feel better.

They are usually positive, upbeat individuals, who have great attitudes and help you to do the same. Then there are those people whose presence feels like a heavy weight on your shoulders. Their negativity spreads like an infectious disease and spending time with them can bring you down and ruin your day. These are the toxic people; people who have a way of sucking the joy right out of your life without even trying.

Exposure to toxic people is like exposure to toxic chemicals; the greater the exposure the more they can make you sick. In the case of toxic people, they make you sick by raising your stress level and all of the negative effects that come with it. Avoid these toxic people as much as you can. There are millions of other people in the world that you can surround yourself with who will contribute to your wellbeing rather than detracting from it. You don't need to compromise your health just to have friends, and it is just as easy to be loved by a positive person as it is by a toxic one.

Toxic people are everywhere. You will run into them at work, in the grocery store and at sporting events. Wherever there are people there will also be toxic people. Do your best to avoid them altogether, to spend as little time with them as possible when you can't avoid them, and to let go of the negative impact they have on you as quickly as you can. Many of the stress management tools in the next chapter can help you do this.

Interactions with toxic strangers can be minimized, but sometimes toxic people are members of your own family that you love dearly. Loving them doesn't make them less toxic, but it does mean that instead of avoiding them, you will have to develop defensive skills in order to deal with them; to minimize their ability to affect your stress level and health. The most important of these skills is remembering that you and only you control your reactions and feelings. In the famous words of Eleanor Roosevelt "No one can make you feel inferior without your consent." So don't consent.

KEEP THINGS IN PERSPECTIVE

Sometimes we perceive things to be far more important than they really are and doing so can lead to unnecessary stress. When we consider things from a broader perspective and remove the emotions which may be attached to them, it becomes easier to clearly evaluate their true importance. Something that might appear to be a crisis worth stressing over or feel like the most important thing in the world may actually seem trivial when viewed in the grand scheme of things. When you find yourself becoming stressed ask yourself, "How important is this, really?" "Will it matter either directly or indirectly a year from now? Ten years from now?" "Is it worth compromising my health for?" Some things are, and some things aren't, and being able to tell the difference is important.

DON'T MAKE TOO MANY CHANGES AT ONCE

Major life changes such as the birth of a baby, the death of a loved one, divorce or changing jobs can be very stressful. Many of these things you have no control over, but if you are anticipating a major change do what you can to limit others. Buying a new home or moving when you are in the process of starting a family or beginning a new career can increase your stress level from manageable to disabling.

14

RELAXATION TECHNIQUES

The mind, the body and your emotions are all interconnected. What affects one affects the others. If your body is
stressed, your mind may be less focused, you will have difficulty concentrating, and your emotions will be less stable. If
your mind is stressed, your body will respond accordingly and
your emotions can run amuck. When practicing relaxation
techniques, it is important to remain aware of your mind and
your body. As you will see, most of the techniques that follow
help you to do just that.

BREATHING

Whenever you begin to feel stressed it is helpful to concentrate on your breathing. Physically it helps to calm your system
and mentally it helps you to regain your composure, focus your
attention, and to think more clearly. Many people find it difficult to control their thoughts when they are frightened, emotionally upset or stressed. Their thoughts become like a
runaway train, filled with speed but unable to reach a destination. Training yourself to be able to take charge of your mind
and redirect your thoughts gives you greater control over how
you respond to stressful situations mentally, and therefore

physically. When you focus carefully on your breathing your mind is unable to wander off and is forced to remain in the present moment, an important aspect of managing stress. This is one of the great advantages of meditation which will be discussed later. It is also why the Lamaze Method, a program based on controlled breathing, is such an effective tool for helping women in labor relax and cope with the pain of childbirth—a very stressful event.

Breathing is an excellent stress reducer that can be done anywhere, any time, and under any conditions. There are many effective breathing techniques. Here are a few simple ones that are easy to learn and easy to do.

The Deep Cleansing Breath

Breathing through your nose, inhale as deeply as you can, completely filling your lungs, then exhale, allowing the lungs to empty fully. Very often, especially when we are nervous or anxious we do not exhale fully, instead rushing to the next breath. This prevents some of the used air from escaping our lungs and reduces the room for new, oxygen rich air to be brought in. Taking deep cleansing breaths frequently throughout the day helps prevent the build up of stress.

The Let it Go Breath

When you become comfortable with the deep cleansing breath you can coordinate it with movements of the head and shoulders to help relieve muscle tension and increase blood flow to your brain. As you exhale completely, allow your chin to fall towards your chest and let your whole body go limp. When you inhale, allow your head to move backwards as if trying to touch the back of your head to the back of your neck. Raise your shoulders towards your ears, then relax them and let your head fall forward and allow your body to go limp again. Strive to create a rhythmic movement in which your breathing defines the pace and your head and neck movements follow its lead. Remember to fill and empty your lungs completely with each breath and to concentrate on the breathing rather than allowing other thoughts to enter your mind. Repeat the sequence several times until you feel the muscles in your neck and shoulders relax. If you feel lightheaded, breathe more slowly or pause and begin again.

The Slow Down Breath

Breathe deliberately and slowly, not necessarily deeply. Continue for at least 2–3 minutes. This technique is very helpful when you find yourself rushing around and needing to slow your pace a bit.

The Distracters: Counted and Patterned Breathing

Counted Breathing

Counting while you breathe helps you to train your mind and concentrate. It can also help you do a better job of both fully expanding and fully emptying your lungs. The more you practice this technique the easier it will become and the longer you will be able to extend the counts. Counted breathing has four stages. Begin by exhaling fully, then, breathe in slowly for a full count of 5 seconds. Hold the breath for 5 seconds, then exhale for a full 5 seconds. If you can, allow your lungs to remain empty for 5 seconds as well. If this is too uncomfortable for you, simply repeat the first three stages until you feel more relaxed. Eventually as the exercises becomes more familiar you can add in the fourth stage. If practiced regularly, you will be able to increase the number of seconds you remain in each stage and breathing more deeply will begin to come naturally.

Patterned Breathing

Like counted breathing, breathing in a rhythmic pattern requires more concentration than simple deep breathing does.

Patterned breathing consists of a series of breaths of different durations. The patterns can be as simple as inhaling in three short, quick parts and exhaling in one long breath, or as complex as the puffing and blowing of Lamaze breathing. You can even breathe in the pattern of a favorite piece of music. What is critical is to always fill and empty your lungs completely and to concentrate on the breathing. Don't allow your mind to wander. This is an exercise in focusing your thoughts as well as a way to release the physical effects of stress.

Breath of Fire

Borrowed from yoga, this technique takes a little practice to master, but it not only increases your oxygen intake and relaxes you, it can give you a mini workout that's great for your abdominal muscles.

When you breathe correctly, your abdomen should expand as you inhale, though many people do just the reverse. When some people take a deep breath, they suck their abdomens in instead of allowing them to expand freely as they should. To begin the Breath of Fire, it is necessary to make sure that your abdomen is moving in the right direction, so go slowly until you can expand on inhalation and contract on exhalation consistently. Place your fingers on your diaphragm to feel that it is moving correctly. Once you have the movement down, while breathing only through your nose, rapidly contract your diaphragm to force short, quick exhalations. You might find it helpful to leave your fingers on your diaphragm as you do this exercise. Each time your diaphragm relaxes your lungs will naturally draw in air, so only focus on the rapid contraction of your diaphragm, exhaling, and making sure that your abdomen is moving in the right direction with each breath. Your goal is to do one-hundred quick breaths in rapid succession, but you can start with twenty-five and build up.

STRETCHING

The simplest way to reduce the tension in your muscles is to stretch them. You should change position and stretch often throughout the day. Some easy stretches that you can do anywhere are:

Gentle Head Rolls

Slowly and gently rotate your head in a circular motion then repeat in the opposite direction until you feel your neck relax.

Shoulder Circles

Lift your shoulders towards your ears then back and down as far as they will comfortably go. Bring them forward and back up to your ears. Repeat in the opposite directions.

Chair Stretch

Clasp your hands behind your chair and stretch backwards to release the tension in your shoulders, arms and chest. Lift one leg and extend it forward as far as you can. Alternate pointing and flexing your toes, then relax and repeat with the other leg.

Trunk Rotations

In a standing position, place your hands on your hips and slowly rotate your body from the waist up in large circles; first one direction and then the other.

Hip Rotations

The same as trunk rotations only this time circle your hips instead.

Jaw Drop and Eyebrow Lift

When your facial muscles become tense, or if you find yourself clenching your teeth, allow your jaw to drop and gently move it from side to side. To release tension in your forehead, raise and lower your eyebrows.

PROGRESSIVE MUSCLE RELAXATION

This technique increases your awareness of your body and encourages you to become mindful of how and where stress is expressing itself in your body. Wherever stress takes up residence, you will find an increase in muscle tension. Common locations are the neck, shoulders and jaw. Sequential contraction and relaxation of your muscles helps release this tension, and the mental focus required to do it correctly helps to elicit the relaxation response.

- Find a comfortable position and close your eyes. This technique can be done sitting or while lying down.
- Contract the muscles of your toes, squeezing tightly and hold for a count of ten. Concentrate on the feeling of tenseness in your toes.
- Release the muscles in your toes and breathe deeply.

Concentrate on the pleasurable sensation of the release.

- Repeat this process moving up the body by contracting, holding, and releasing each muscle group one at a time.
- Include all major muscle groups; your calves, thighs, buttocks, abdomen, hands, upper arms, shoulders, neck and face.

MEDITATION

Meditation is a practice that when done regularly gives you the ability to control the activity of your mind and your emotions the same way you control the movements of your body. Have you ever had a song stuck in your head that just kept playing over and over again and you couldn't get it to stop? You couldn't control your mind because you have probably never been trained to do so. Being able to control the mind may seem a strange concept in western culture but it has been a part of eastern culture for thousands of years.

Dr. Herbert Benson of the Harvard Medical School studied eastern mystics extensively in order to better understand their amazing abilities. Few of us could ever hope to accomplish a level of proficiency in controlling our minds and bodies equal to that of mystics who have spent a lifetime in training, but further research by Dr. Benson was able to reproduce many of the health benefits associated with their practices through the use of simple meditative techniques. His research also demonstrated that meditation does not have to involve any religious or spiritual connotation in order to be effective. Whether or not meditation is used as a spiritual endeavor is up to the individual. Its primary value in stress management is as an efficient method for training the mind and bringing it under your control. This gives you the power to prevent a great deal of stress and an effective way to elicit the relaxation response when it is needed.

There are many approaches to meditation and I encourage you to investigate different methods to find one that works for you and that you are comfortable with. Personally, I have found great value in a method described in the book, *Meditation, A simple 8- point program for translating spiritual ideals into daily life* by Eknath Easwaran, but there are many alternatives from which to choose.

Most forms of meditation share at least two common elements. The first is the silent repetition of a word or a phrase called a mantra, or the silent reciting of an inspirational passage. The mantra can be any word or phase of your choosing. Words such as "peace" or "relax" are common, as is the use of religious words and phrases such as "Jesus," "Allah," "Shalom," "Rama," or "Hail, Mary full of grace."

The second element is the focusing of your attention on the sound of your mantra or passage and nothing else. When other thoughts drift into your mind, ignore them. Giving them your attention increases their importance. If someone arrives late to a meeting but his or her entrance is disregarded by the others in the room, the meeting won't be disrupted much. But if everyone stops what they are doing and turns their attention to the late comer, the disruption of the meeting will be much greater. It is the same with invading thoughts. They are inevitable at first, but rather than paying attention to them, disregard them and attempt to return your attention to your mantra or passage.

Meditation is most effective when it is practiced regularly. Just twenty or thirty minutes once or twice a day can have a tremendous impact on your overall wellbeing. To get the most from your practice of meditation:

- Create a space that is comfortable for you to meditate in. It should be a quiet location with a comfortable chair or cushion to sit on, and any items that may encourage you to relax such as a plant, personal mementos, or items of spiritual significance. Meditating in a garden, at the beach, or anywhere outdoors is wonderful if you can find a quiet place away from traffic and interruptions where you feel comfortable and safe.
- Sit in a comfortable position with your eyes closed. Sitting is preferred to lying down because once you become relaxed, it is easy to fall asleep.
- Breathe deliberately and slowly, taking several deep cleansing breaths.
- Begin saying your mantra or passage silently to yourself.
- When other thoughts drift into your head, ignore them and return to your mantra or passage.
- Don't judge yourself. Meditation is not a contest or a challenge.

Meditating for as little as ten minutes can be effective, but twenty to thirty minutes will give your body a greater opportunity to take advantage of the relaxation response. When you are finished meditating, slowly allow awareness of your body and your surroundings to return and open your eyes. Rest a moment and take a few more deep cleansing breaths before you try to move.

The more regularly you practice meditation, the easier it will become. As with any form of training, over time your body will become conditioned to meditating and will respond by initiating the relaxation response more quickly. You will also find that with regular practice you are better able to redirect your thoughts at will. When negative or stressful ideas and emotions fill your mind, you can refocus your attention onto your mantra or onto more positive and productive thoughts. You may even be able to stop that song from playing in your head!

YOGA

Yoga incorporates exercise, controlled breathing, and meditation all into one practice making it one of the best stress reducing options available. As a form of exercise, Yoga is wonderful. It incorporates all three elements of physical fitness—strength, endurance and flexibility—and leaves you feeling relaxed, yet energized. It can be practiced at any level of fitness, and by everyone from the very young to the very old, and even the very pregnant. Yoga results in total conditioning of the body as well as enhancing your mental focus and concentration. Through meditation, yoga helps raise the mind above the difficulties of life and improves your mental outlook. For some practitioners, it provides a spiritual experience helping them to feel more connected to themselves and to the universe around them, and it becomes their way of life.

Practicing yoga involves breathing techniques and a series of stretches and physical postures or poses known as asanas, designed to exercise the body and calm the mind. And no, you don't have to be a contortionist to participate. While very advanced students may assume positions that resemble human pretzels, everyone can experience tremendous benefits from practicing yoga regardless of how strong or flexible they are — or aren't!

There are many styles of yoga and many approaches to teaching them. Some classes are very gentle, others more vigorous. Yoga may be performed to music, with chanting, or in silence, and with or without the aid of simple equipment. If your experience with one class or one teacher isn't what you had hoped for, try another until you find one that works for you.

PRAYER

Prayer, like meditation helps to focus your mind which helps you to feel calmer. It can be an outlet for anxiety in difficult times, helping to reduce feelings of fear, loneliness and isolation. Patients who pray regularly have been shown to heal faster and cope more effectively with serious illnesses. Believing in, and communicating with a power greater than yourself can be a great source of comfort and peace.

USE YOUR IMAGINATION

Visualization is a purely mental technique that can cause a very physical response; the relaxation response.

- Find a comfortable position and close your eyes.
- Take several deep cleansing breaths.
- Visualize a place that is calm and serene where you would enjoy being. It can be a place that you have experienced in real life that you associate with being calm and happy, or a place entirely of your own imagining.
- Mentally experience this place in as much detail as you can. Concentrate on what this place looks like. What time of year is it? Is it morning, afternoon or evening? What is the weather like? Is it hot or cold? What color is the sky? What else can you see? What do you see if you look to the right? To the left? What does the air or the sun feel like on your face? What do you smell? Rain? Flowers? The scent of the ocean? What do you hear? Are there soothing sounds or the sounds of silence? Now imagine yourself in this place.

Know that you are safe and calm here. Focus on how you feel here. In this place you are relaxed, peaceful and happy.
- Remain in this place as long as you need to in order to feel calm, then, slowly return to reality.
- Take several deep breaths and open your eyes.

I find imagery an especially effective tool when I am somewhere I would prefer not to be. When I am in a stressful place or situation like at the dentist's office or on a flight that is experiencing turbulence, being able to transport myself to a place where I feel safe and calm is wonderful. Like all of the relaxation techniques, imagery and visualization skills improve and become more effective with regular practice.

TAKE A WARM BATH

Surrounding yourself in warm water relaxes your muscles and the sound of running water can wash away your cares. A warm bath can be combined with visualization to increase the effects of each.

AROMATHERAPY

Olfactory stimulation of the brain through the use of perfumed plants and essential oils is another ancient technique that has been rediscovered in modern times. Scents can have a profound affect on the mind and the body. Think about how you react to the smell of baking bread or the scent of a cologne worn by someone you have found attractive. One can stimulate your appetite even if you aren't hungry, and both may trigger fond memories. Essential oils can be used to relieve stress in a variety of ways, but the safest way for home use is to add a few drops of chamomile, bergamot, sandalwood, lavender or sweet marjoram oil to a warm bath. Adding a few drops to a diffuser or a handkerchief and inhaling it periodically is also effective. The use of essential oils is a wonderful addition to a professional massage.

HAVE A MASSAGE

Human touch is a primal need as necessary for health and wellness as food, exercise and sleep. Without touching, children fail to thrive and develop normally, and older adults become depressed and lonely. Of late, American culture has become almost "touchaphobic." With law suits abounding over sexual harassment and sexual abuse in schools, churches, and workplaces, people have become fearful that any touch or physical contact might be misinterpreted so they simply don't touch at all. Teachers rarely hug students, even very young ones, and children are given careful instructions inside the classroom and by parents not to let anyone touch them. In the workplace, anything more than a handshake has become suspect.

We may be becoming a less physically affectionate, more non-tactile society, but biologically the need for touch remains. At Miami's Touch Research Institute, researchers have established that massage can have positive effects on everything from diabetes to migraines, from improving mental clarity to enhancing physical performance, but most especially on reversing the negative effects of stress. Massage boosts the functioning of the immune system and lowers the levels of the stress hormones cortisol and norepinephrine. It improves digestion and stimulates the brain to produce endorphins, those feel good hormones that elevate mood, suppress pain and trigger the relaxation response. Basically, everything negative that stress can do to your body, massage therapy can undo.

There are many styles of massage therapy available, from Swedish to Shiatsu. Some are gentler, others more aggressive, but all are effective in reducing the effects of stress. A full body massage is ideal, but a chair massage that focuses on your upper back, shoulders and neck can be a great way to experience quick relief from stress when you don't have much time or if you prefer not to remove your clothing. Massaging of the hands and feet is also a relaxing experience. Whether you enlist the hands of a friend or family member, or seek the skills of a licensed massage therapist, try to make massage a regular part of your life.

TAKE TIME TO RELAX

It's OK to take time off. The world won't come to an end without you. Go for a walk, read a book, listen to music, play a game, or pursue a hobby—do whatever you enjoy and find relaxing. If you think you can't take time to relax, consider this: If you *don't* take the time to take care of your health, you *will* get sick, and then you will *have to* take the time to get well. Either way you will end up taking the time, but if you wait until you are forced to you may end up taking even more time and you won't get to enjoy it as much.

STRIVE FOR BALANCE

If you work hard, play hard. If you have an exciting job choose leisure activities that are calm, like painting or gardening. If you sit at a desk and think all day, balance your life with physical activity in the evening and vice versa.

Let It All Hang Out

No matter how hard you try, your emotions will not be denied. Attempting to suppress or ignore them is futile because they will eventually surface on their own in the form or poor health or dis-ease. Suppressing or denying your emotions is very unhealthy for your mind and your body; bottled up feelings increase your stress level considerably. Not being able or willing to express your thoughts and emotions also makes it difficult to build open, honest, and healthy relationships, and poor quality relationships will only increase your stress level further.

Allow your emotions an outlet. If you feel like crying, cry. Crying can often communicate in ways that words cannot and it provides a means for both emotional release and the lowering of your body's level of stress hormones. Unlike tears that flow when your eyes are irritated, tears of emotion contain varying levels of stress hormones. They literally help to wash your stress away.

Laugh :~)

Laughter may indeed be the best medicine when it comes to reducing stress related illness. Maintaining a sense of humor and not taking life too seriously lessens the amount of stress you will experience, and a good hard belly laugh can dissipate the effects of stress quickly. Create opportunities for humor in your day wherever you can. I use a daily planner filled with entertaining cartoons that helps me to smile as I consider the demands of the day ahead, and I have jokes on my computer to provide some much needed relief while I work.

If you've had a rough day, instead of watching the evening news which is filled with stressful information and images, watch a funny movie. It will help you to unwind and get a better night's sleep.

SOCIALIZE

Just as physical human contact is necessary, so is social interaction and emotional support. In the famous words of John Donne, "No man is an island." Spend time with loved ones and friends that bring you joy. Having a network of people who you care about and who are supportive of you can go a long way towards making life less stressful. Positive experiences are more enjoyable and the burden of difficult times and challenges is eased when you have others to share them with.

GET A PET

Having a pet may be even more comforting for stressed individuals than the support of people. Pets are almost always happy to see you, they offer unconditional love, and they are nonjudgmental. Research has shown that pet owners have lower heart rates and blood pressure during stressful events than non-pet owners and they are more likely to survive a heart attack.

PERFORM A RANDOM ACT OF KINDNESS

Doing something for someone else also does something for you: it relieves stress. When we remain caught up in our own lives, it's difficult to keep things in perspective. When we reach out to others it makes us feel good about ourselves and helps to shift the focus away from our own problems. People who do for others are generally happier and more relaxed than people who don't.

Don't Manage Stress Through the Use of Drugs, Alcohol or Cigarettes!

An occasional drink can help you to relax and may have some health benefits, but regular use of alcohol, recreational drugs or cigarettes to cope with stress is dangerous. All three negatively impact your health and can easily become addictive.

IV. SLEEP

15

RECHARGING YOUR BATTERIES

Getting sufficient rest each day is just as important to good health as eating right, getting enough exercise, and managing stress. It affects your body's strength, your mind's ability to think, and your emotional stability. During sleep is when your body performs most of its routine maintenance. This is the time when your body uses the raw materials you have supplied it with throughout the day to rebuild or replace damaged or worn out tissue, and to build new tissue. Sleep provides the down time that your body and mind need to recuperate from the stresses of life and to prepare to meet the challenges of tomorrow.

The amount of time American's spend sleeping has steadily declined from an average of nine hours at the beginning of the twentieth century to about seven and a half hours at the beginning of the twenty-first. Millions of Americans are routinely getting by on less than six hours of sleep. Many even view surviving on less sleep as a symbol of their strength or dedication, wearing their exhaustion like a badge of honor. However, sleep deprivation is reaching epidemic proportions and may soon be our nation's number one health problem.

While there are variations in how much sleep an individual

needs, studies show that most people need *at least* eight hours a night for optimum health and performance, with many people needing nine or ten to feel their best. If you don't get the sleep you need, you will develop a sleep debt that must be repaid one way or another; there is no cheating Mother Nature. Some people truly believe that they can get by on less sleep without suffering any serious consequences or impairing their performance, but most are mistaken. Research has shown that sleep deprived people can't be relied upon to accurately judge their own performance capabilities. They may feel as if they are only slightly sleepy when in fact their ability to function physically and psychologically is at its lowest level. This misperception can lead to a false sense of security and result in compromised health and safety. Some people pay off their sleep debt by sleeping longer on the weekend or taking naps, but sadly others pay it off with their health or even their lives.

When you don't get enough sleep you are more likely to suffer from certain chronic illnesses, including diabetes and heart disease. You are also more likely to gain weight or become obese. An otherwise healthy person's capacity to process blood sugar may be reduced by as much as 30% when they are sleep deprived.

Sleep deprivation disrupts your body's ability to manage glucose and can make your cells more resistant to insulin. If you recall from the EAT section, insulin resistance causes your cells to think they are starving even though there is plenty of sugar in your blood. They send a message to your brain which triggers hunger, encouraging you to eat more. You don't metabolize the additional carbohydrates you consume properly, so you end up storing the extra intake as fat. The more fat you store, the more weight you gain, and the more insulin resistant you are likely to become. Two other hormones which are important in the regulation of appetite, energy balance, and obesity—leptin and ghrelin—are also affected by sleep.

It might sound logical that the busier you are and the less sleep you get the more calories you would burn and therefore the more weight you would lose, but in fact, it has just the opposite effect. Due to these disturbances in your metabolism, not getting enough sleep can cause you to gain weight. The extra weight further increases your risk for diabetes, heart disease and other illnesses.

Sleep deprivation also increases levels of the stress hormone cortisol. As you discovered in the RELAX section, the effects of elevated stress hormones are very destructive to both your physical health and your mental wellbeing. They can suppress your immune system, increase your risk of chronic disease, impair you memory and lead to depression. When you are overtired, everything becomes more difficult and even simple challenges can become stressful events. Mood seems to be especially sensitive to not getting enough sleep. Overtired people tend to be more irritable and experience more anger, anxiety and sadness. They also have a lower sex drive. The bottom line is that when you don't get enough sleep you can't think as clearly, accomplish as much, cope as well, or enjoy anything as fully as when you are well rested.

People who sleep fewer than six hours a night don't live as long as people who sleep seven hours or more. They not only suffer from more chronic illnesses but are also injured in more accidents. Drowsy driving and falling asleep at the wheel have become a devastating problem on America's roadways resulting in thousands of injuries and deaths each year.

Being awake for more than 18 to 24 hours can reduce your

alertness and performance as much as having a blood-alcohol concentration of .05 to .10 (in many states the definition of legally drunk is .08) seriously impairing your ability to drive. Some people also experience something known as Automatic Behavior Syndrome where part of the brain goes to sleep while other parts continue working. If you have ever been driving down the road and suddenly realized that you aren't sure where you are, you have probably experienced this phenomenon. Your conscious brain took a short nap while the rest of you continued driving on autopilot. Unfortunately, your autopilot isn't designed to respond to the unexpected or to prevent accidents. Most states can charge you with causing a crash or a fatality after falling asleep at the wheel, but in July of 2003, New Jersey passed a bill known as "Maggie's Law" which is the first law in the country to establish fatigued driving as "recklessness" under the vehicular homicide statute. Other states are expected to pass similar bills in the future. Hopefully with enough increased awareness, the public will come to understand that driving while sleep deprived is as dangerous as driving under the influence of drugs or alcohol.

UNDERSTANDING SLEEP

In preparation for sleep your body secretes the hormone melatonin and your body becomes more relaxed. You begin to breathe more slowly and your body temperature falls slightly. There are two phases of sleep. The first known as non-REM (Rapid Eye Movement) sleep or "quiet sleep" consists of four stages. This phase is followed by a period of REM sleep which is characterized by the eyes moving rapidly behind closed lids, and an increase in heart rate, breathing and metabolism. REM sleep is when dreaming takes place and it can last anywhere from ten to forty minutes. When REM sleep is complete, the body returns to non-REM sleep and the process repeats itself. This happens several times a night.

As you enter the first stage of non-REM sleep your brain waves change from rapid beta waves to slower alpha waves, then theta waves and eventually they slow all the way down to delta waves. Delta sleep is the deepest sleep and the most restorative. It takes most people between seventy to ninety minutes to reach delta sleep and anything that interferes with the earlier stages of non-REM sleep may prevent them from reaching it at all. When sleep is interrupted, the body must start over again, it can't just pick up where it left off. If your sleep is frequently interrupted it can leave you feeling tired and irritable instead of refreshed, and your body won't be able to heal or repair itself as well.

WHY PEOPLE DON'T GET ENOUGH SLEEP

There are numerous reasons why people don't get enough sleep. As mentioned earlier, many people just don't grasp that they aren't getting enough. They have been overtired so long and have developed enough coping mechanisms to deal with sleep deprivation that they have come to believe that how they feel is normal. They don't realize that they could feel and function much better than they currently are. If you want to know if you are getting enough sleep, answer the following questions:

- Do you have difficulty waking up in the morning or often wake up feeling like you could have slept longer?
- In order to get going in the morning do you need to jump start your day with a stimulant like caffeine?
- Do you feel sleepy or find yourself dozing off while you are watching TV or reading a book?

- How about when you are sitting in a meeting or in traffic?
- Are you easily fatigued or feel like you react more slowly than you should?
- Do you find it difficult to concentrate or listen when someone is speaking or to understand directions?
- Do you have difficulty thinking or remembering information?
- Do you make frequent errors or mistakes at work or in going about your daily activities?
- Do you often become impatient or easily angered?
- Are you frequently irritable, sad or depressed?
- Do you have problems with your eyes burning or focusing?
- Have you been gaining weight even though you are eating well and getting enough exercise?

If you answered yes to one or more of these questions there is a good chance that you aren't getting all the sleep you need. A person who is fully rested and has gotten adequate sleep wakes up easily feeling refreshed, alert, and in good spirits, and they are able to function well throughout the day without the aid of chemical stimulants. Some medications may cause you to feel as if you haven't had enough sleep, but if you aren't taking anything that should make you feel less alert, you are most likely feeling the affects of a sleep debt. If you aren't getting enough sleep there could be several reasons why:

You Choose Not To

Many people selectively deprive themselves of sleep in favor of social activities. Even though they know it will leave them tired in the morning, they stay up to watch a favorite show, go out with friends, or enjoy some form of entertainment.

To Improve Performance

Many students pass on sleep trying to cram for exams. "Pulling an all-nighter" is a common practice, but not a very productive one since being overtired makes it more difficult to concentrate and retain information. Working long hours to compete more effectively in the workplace is also a common obstacle to getting enough sleep that is counterproductive. Sacrificing your sleep to attain your goals usually ends up compromising your health instead.

Your Lifestyle

Smoking, poor diet, lack of exercise, alcohol consumption and caffeine use can all interfere with your ability to get a good night's sleep.

You Are Too Stressed to Sleep

Worrying and an overactive brain can sometimes make it almost impossible to get to sleep. There are many ways to help you regain control over your stress responses in the RELAX section as well as some sleep specific ideas in the next chapter.

A Poor Sleep Environment

An uncomfortable or worn out mattress, too much light, noise, or not enough humidity can interfere with your sleep. So can sleeping in a room that's too warm or one that is filled with distractions.

Shift Work

We have become a twenty-four hour a day society. Shift work used to be an issue for miners, health care, and emergency workers but now it is pervasive throughout the workplace from grocery stores to manufacturing.

Traveling Across Time Zones

We have also become a very mobile society. Frequent flyers who travel long distances often have trouble keeping their bodies in sync with their location. This can easily disrupt sleep.

Menopause

The hormonal fluctuations of menopause can disrupt sleep in several ways, especially via hot flashes that occur in the middle of the night. Try including more soy products and omega-3 fatty acids in your diet, or talk with your health care professional. There are many wonderful books available that can help you get through the change more easily.

Medications

Many medications, both over the counter ones and prescription ones, can interfere with sleep. Talk to your doctor or pharmacist to see if the drugs you are using could be the source of your sleep difficulties. They may be able to recommend alternatives.

RESETTING YOUR BIOLOGICAL CLOCK

All humans have an inborn biological clock that regulates body processes including sleep known as the circadian rhythm. These circadian rhythms control normal fluctuations in body temperature and hormone production that tell your body when to sleep and when to wake up. If you travel across time zones or work shift work, your circadian rhythms become out of sync with your environment causing you to feel tired, uncomfortable and experience all of the symptoms commonly referred to as jet lag. You can minimize the amount of jet lag you experience and speed up the resetting of your biological clock by following some simple strategies.

Get as much exposure to sunlight as possible. Sunlight helps to reset the circadian rhythms, so when you travel spend as much time outdoors during the day as you can. The more hours of exposure to sunlight your body receives, the faster your clock will reset.

Schedule your travel so as to arrive in the early evening local time and stay up until at least 10 p.m.

Plan ahead. Go to bed and get up earlier for several days prior to traveling eastward, and later when traveling westward. Your body adapts better to going backwards rather than forwards which is why you experience more jet lag when traveling east than when traveling west.

Avoid alcohol, caffeine and heavy exercise before bedtime.

Melatonin supplements. Melatonin is a hormone that your body produces to help induce sleep. Studies have shown that taking melatonin as a dietary supplement before bed can help to reset the biological clock quickly, but there is insufficient research available to recommend the correct dosage, the correct time to take the supplement, or to determine what the long term affects might be. Hormones are powerful biological agents and should be used with great caution. Talk to your health care professional before using this product.

Keeping a Sleep Diary

If you are having trouble sleeping, you may find it helpful to keep a sleep diary. Each day record what time you went to bed, how long it took you to fall asleep, how many times you woke up during the night, how long you slept, and what time you woke up in the morning. Make a note of how you feel when you wake up and throughout the day and compare it with the checklist on page 171. Also keep track of how much caffeine you consumed and when, how much exercise you got, how much alcohol you drank, any medications you took, and what you did right before you went to bed. Reviewing your sleep diary may help you determine why you are having problems with your sleep. It is also a good tool for communicating with your health care professional. The National Sleep Foundation has a free diary that includes all of the necessary information available on line at *www.sleepfoundation.org*.

16

GETTING A GOOD NIGHT'S SLEEP

Most people who suffer from general insomnia can improve the quality of their sleep by making healthier lifestyle choices such as going to bed instead of staying up late, getting more exercise or drinking less alcohol. Because everything to do with your health is so interconnected, whatever you do to improve your overall wellness will likely improve your sleep also, and vice versa. If you make a genuine effort to get enough high quality sleep, you will have more energy to exercise with and be better able to manage stress. The more exercise you get and the better you manage your stress, the better you will sleep. The most important thing is to make a beginning, and getting a good night's sleep is a wonderful place to start.

There are several things that you can to do to improve your sleep. The first of course is to recognize how important it is to the wellbeing of your mind and your body and to determine how much sleep you need. The general recommendation is that most people need at least eight hours, but sleep requirements vary greatly between individuals. One way to determine how much sleep you need is to pay attention to how many hours you sleep when you have the option of sleeping as much as you want to.

If you are sleeping many more hours on the weekend than during the week, you are obviously not getting enough sleep during the week and your body is using the weekend to repay its sleep debt. Increase the number of hours you sleep during the week until you find that you are waking up at the same time on Saturday and Sunday as you do in the middle of the week. This will be an indication that you are no longer incurring a sleep debt. You can also do this during a vacation if you have enough time off and aren't staying up late or drinking more alcohol than normal. For the first few days of a vacation you will probably be paying back on your sleep debt, but by the end of a week you should be caught up and sleeping the number of hours your body actually needs. Everyday life is usually more stressed filled than vacation time, and stress increases your need for sleep, so your sleep requirements are likely to be a little higher when you return to normal activities, but at least you will have an estimate of how much sleep your body needs and a place to begin. You can also keep a sleep diary that includes how much sleep you get each night and how you feel the following day. Many people are surprised to find that they need more than they thought.

Once you know how much sleep you need, make getting a good night's sleep as much of a priority in your life as your family and your work are. Taking enough time to rest isn't being lazy or selfish, it's just the opposite. The more rested you are the more effective you will be both in personal relationships and on the job. Sleep deprivation costs American businesses billions of dollars in lost productivity and accident related expenses each year.

The DOs and DON'Ts of Getting a Great Night's Sleep

The DOs

Do Try to Go to Bed and Wake Up at the Same Time Everyday

Sleeping late on a Sunday morning may sound like a wonderful thing to do, and it is a good way to pay off some of your sleep debt, but if you sleep too long, it may make it harder to get to sleep on Sunday night. Your body responds best to consistent routines and it will become conditioned to fall asleep at certain times if you stick to a regular sleep and wake routine. Besides, if you start getting enough sleep during the week, you won't need the extra sleep on the weekend and you can use those morning hours to do something you enjoy.

Do Eat Right

Following the healthy eating guidelines in this manual will help to stabilize your blood sugar level, keeping you more comfortable during the night. Remember that a healthy bedtime snack is important. A small bowl of cereal with milk or soy milk, a slice of whole wheat bread with peanut butter and banana slices, half a turkey sandwich or a low-fat yogurt that isn't too high in sugar are good choices.

Do Get Enough Exercise

It provides an outlet for stress, reduces the effects of the 'fight or flight' response, and stimulates the relaxation response. A lower body temperature signals your body that it's time to sleep, so don't build up lots of heat in your body by exercising too close to bedtime. Exercising late is better than not exercising at all, but try to finish your exercise at least three hours before you plan to go to sleep.

Do Give Your Mind a Chance to Relax

Take a break from stimulating activities and give your brain some time to relax before trying to fall asleep. If you engage in challenging mental activity right before bed, it will be more difficult for your mind to let go and rest. You can condition your brain to relax by creating bedtime rituals that signal the day is done like taking a hot bath, reading, listening to calming music, or having a cup of soothing herbal tea. If you do the same thing every night right before bed, both your body and mind will learn to respond to the ritual by gearing down for sleep.

Do Clear Your Mind of Concerns

As part of your bedtime ritual, take a few minutes each evening to organize what you need to do the next day and write it down. The less you have to keep track of in your mind when you are trying to fall asleep, the better. It will also give you peace of mind that important matters won't be forgotten. This practice also works well if you are concerned about something. Writing it down along with any ideas you have for addressing it is a way to express your feelings and let go of stress.

Do Get as Much Exposure to Natural Light as Possible

Sunlight helps to keep your body's clock running on time and can help reduce depression. If you work indoors, try to spend your lunch hour and breaks outside or at least near a sunny window.

Do Create a Comfortable Environment for Sleeping

The place where you sleep should be designed for sleeping and sex, not for working or other activities.

- **Light:** The room should be dark. Cover windows with blackout curtains or darkening shades. If necessary, wear eye shades to keep out extra light. If you need a night light for safety, make sure that it isn't too bright.
- **Sound:** Noise is disruptive to sleep so make your sleep area as quiet as possible. "White noise" created by a sound device, a fan, or a fountain can help to drown out other more disturbing sounds. If you sleep with a partner who snores, see the snoring section in the next chapter for suggestions. If all else fails, wear earplugs that reduce noise, but not ones that block all noise. It is important that you be able to hear emergency sounds like a smoke or fire alarm.
- **Temperature:** Keep your sleeping space cool. The room temperature should be set wherever you are most comfortable. For most people that is between 65 and 75 degrees Fahrenheit.
- **Humidity:** Air that is too dry can cause your nasal passages to become dry and increase snoring. Use a humidifier if necessary.
- **Comfort:** You will spend about 3,000 hours in your bed this year so be sure you have a comfortable mattress. Most mattresses need to be replaced every 8 -10 years. Pillows should support your head but not flex your neck. 100% cotton sheets with long fibers and higher thread counts are much more comfortable than cotton synthetic blends. They are worth their added cost for the comfort alone, but they will also last longer. Blankets and comforters should be the

correct weight for the climate you live in. You should be cool enough to sleep but warm enough that you don't have to curl up to conserve body warmth. Also make sure that your bed is large enough for you to move around freely.

- **Color:** Decorate your sleep space in calming colors like blues, greens, violets or browns.
- **Safety:** Remove or secure obstacles like electrical cords that you might trip or fall over in the darkness.
- **Distractions:** Remove anything that stimulates you and replace it with things that calm you. If being able to see a clock keeps you awake, face it away from you or place it behind a picture of someone you love or a vase of flowers. Artwork should be calming, not stimulating.

DON'Ts

Don't Consume Too Much Caffeine

Some people are more affected by caffeine than others, and there is a great deal of variation in how quickly a person's body processes it. Most people only feel the effects of caffeine for three to five hours, but for others it can remain in their systems for up to twelve hours. Try to avoid consuming products containing caffeine such as coffee, tea, soft drinks and chocolate several hours before bedtime.

Don't Smoke!

Like caffeine, nicotine is a stimulant. It is also addictive, so heavy smokers experience withdrawal symptoms during the night which can disrupt their sleep. Some smokers think that having a cigarette before bed will relax them and help them to sleep, but that is not the case. The ritual of smoking may be a relaxing activity, but the chemicals you inhale actually impair your ability to sleep.

Don't Drink Too Close to Bedtime

Alcohol may have a sedative affect and can help you to relax, but it may have a rebound affect that can cause you to wake suddenly in the middle of the night. It also makes it more difficult for your body to reach the deeper, restorative stages of sleep. Drinking too much of anything too close to bedtime can result in a full bladder requiring you to wake up to use the bathroom.

Don't Go to Bed on a Full Stomach

A light snack can help you sleep better but a heavy meal or lots of spicy food in your stomach at bedtime can lead to heartburn.

Don't Stay in Bed When You Can't Sleep

If you can't fall asleep right away, don't just lie there. Get up and go do something until you feel drowsy again.

Don't Stress Over the Fact That You Aren't Falling Asleep

Checking the clock every few minutes to see how much later it is will only give you one more thing to worry about, increase your stress hormone levels, and make it more difficult for you to fall asleep. Instead, focus on something calming, like the mantra you use for meditation or the sound of your breathing. If there is something in particular keeping you awake, get up and write it down. You can address it tomorrow when you are rested enough to deal with it effectively, rather than letting your mind waste precious sleep time worrying about it while you are tired and less likely to come up with an effective solution.

Don't Watch Stimulating Programs Right Before it's Time to Sleep

Watching TV or a movie too close to bedtime can make it difficult to get to sleep, especially if the program is exciting or frightening. Even the evening news is usually filled with distressing images and information that can stimulate your brain and emotions. If you do watch a program before going to bed, choose something that is calming and won't send your brain or emotions into overdrive.

Don't Work in Your Sleep Area

Having a desk, a computer or anything else in your bedroom that acts as a constant reminder of things you have to do can make it difficult for your mind to let go and relax. Your bed and your bedroom should be a place for sleep and sex and nothing else.

WHAT ABOUT NAPPING?

Taking a power nap can help reduce your sleep debt and be a great pick me in the middle of the afternoon. In many parts of the world a mid-afternoon break or siesta is standard practice and with good reason. It's not only the hottest part of the day; it's also when your energy level and body temperature drop as part of your normal circadian rhythms. Even a 15–20 minute nap can boost your energy significantly. If you are going to nap, don't sleep more than an hour. Sleeping longer can leave you feeling groggy. Also try not to nap before noon or after four P.M.; it can make it difficult for you to fall asleep at night.

17

SLEEP DISORDERS

General insomnia or an inability to sleep is usually caused by one of the factors reviewed in the last chapter, but some people suffer from more serious types of sleep disorders. They include loud or excessive snoring, sleep apnea, restless leg syndrome and narcolepsy. All of these disorders can impair your ability to get a good night's rest, but some of them are particularly damaging to your overall health. If you believe that you suffer from a sleep disorder, speak with your health care professional to discuss possible solutions.

SNORING

Just as the muscles in the rest of your body relax when you fall asleep, so do the muscles in your throat. As air passes over these relaxed muscles it can cause them to vibrate creating the familiar sounds of snoring. Snoring can also be caused by being overweight or having a very large neck, allergies, asthma, and nasal deformities as well as smoking and alcohol consumption. Simple snoring isn't a concern if it isn't disturbing your sleep or anyone else's, but it can also be a symptom of sleep apnea, a serious condition that requires medical intervention.

If you are having trouble with snoring, and you are

overweight, losing weight may be the answer. If you smoke, quit. Cut back on alcohol consumption, especially late in the evening. Sleeping on your side instead of on your back and using nasal breathing strips to open up your nasal passages can be very helpful. There are also dental appliances that can be useful. If the problem persists see your health care professional, he or she will probably want to check for sleep apnea.

SLEEP APNEA

Sleep apnea is a serious, potentially life-threatening condition characterized by brief interruptions of breathing during sleep. These interruptions occur when the upper airway becomes completely or partially blocked. Sleep apnea may be associated with irregular heartbeat, high blood pressure, heart attack, and stroke. This condition is far more common than once thought, and is estimated to affect as a many as eighteen million Americans. It is most common in people who snore loudly, are overweight, or have some physical abnormality in the nose, throat or upper airways. The frequent interruptions in airflow can prevent the sufferer from getting enough restorative deep sleep resulting in severe daytime sleepiness. If you suspect that you or someone you know may have sleep apnea, it is important to seek medical attention.

RESTLESS LEG SYNDROME

Restless Leg Syndrome or RLS is just what it sounds like— legs that don't relax and settle down for the night when the rest of you does. People with RLS experience tingling, crawling sensations, or cramping in the legs when they are trying to sleep. To relieve the discomfort most people need to move or stretch their legs, which of course interrupts their sleep and leaves them feeling tired the next day. RLS can be caused by many things including vitamin and mineral deficiencies, medications, problems with the kidneys or diabetes. RLS seems to run in families suggesting that it might be a hereditary condition. If you suffer from RLS talk to your health care professional.

NARCOLEPSY

Narcolepsy is another condition that requires medical intervention. People who suffer from narcolepsy are often extremely tired during the day and go though periods of unexpected sleep or the overwhelming need to sleep. They may sometimes experience a sudden loss of muscle control, be unable to talk or move briefly when falling asleep or waking up, or spend a lot of time operating on autopilot not fully aware or able to remember what they are doing.

PART TWO:

IMPORTANT SAFETY PRECAUTIONS

Eating right, exercising, managing stress, and getting enough sleep are important things to do, but sometimes what not to do is just as important to your health. Minimizing your exposure to harmful substances such as tobacco, drugs and alcohol, as well as those found in your environment and your food, can go a long way towards improving the quality of your health and your life. We live in a world fraught with danger and hazards. Being exposed to diseases, extreme weather conditions, or simply riding in a car can have serious consequence if you don't take the necessary steps to protect yourself.

18

SAFER SEX

There are over twenty different forms of sexually transmitted diseases (STD). Some like syphilis are curable, others like AIDS are not. I use the term "safer" rather than "safe" for good reason. In the words of the Center for Disease Control:

"The surest way to avoid transmission of sexually transmitted diseases is to abstain from sexual intercourse, or to be in a long-term mutually monogamous relationship with a partner who has been tested and you know is uninfected."

"For persons whose sexual behaviors place them at risk for STDs, correct and consistent use of the male latex condom can reduce the risk of STD transmission. **However, no protective method is 100 percent effective, and condom use cannot guarantee absolute protection against any STD."**

Condoms offer a measure of protection against STD's, but condoms can be used incorrectly, they can break, they are damaged by the use of oil-based lubricants such as petroleum jelly, and they don't cover all parts of the body that can transmit disease. Genital ulcer diseases such as genital herpes, syphilis and chancroid are transmitted via skin-to-skin contact rather than through body fluids. If your partner has sores anywhere that your skin can come in contact with such as the scrotum or anus, a condom will not be effective in protecting you against infection. If you are going to have sex with anyone other than a mutually monogamous partner, ***always*** use a condom, but realize that you are still putting yourself at risk. The best way to prevent STD's is to:

- Avoid casual sex with people you don't know well.
- Avoid sexual contact with anyone who has genital or anal sores, a rash, discharge or any other sign of venereal disease.
- Know how to use a condom correctly and use it consistently.
- Don't use petroleum based lubricants with latex condoms.

Sexually transmitted diseases including AIDS cannot be contracted through casual physical contact such as shaking hands or by coming in contact with toilet seats, telephones, dishes or other objects. Most organisms that cause sexually transmitted diseases usually die within a minute outside the body. AIDS and syphilis can be contracted through blood to blood contact such as the sharing of IV needles. You ***cannot*** get AIDS from donating blood. If you suspect that you may have been infected with any STD refrain from having sexual contact with others and seek medical attention.

19

TOBACCO PRODUCTS

Since the first Surgeon General's Report on the health consequences of smoking in 1964, we have been aware of the negative effects this activity has on the body. In the almost forty years since, the case against all tobacco products has strengthened tremendously. There is probably no other single activity other than driving while intoxicated that puts your health and wellbeing at as much risk as does the use of tobacco products. Cigarette smoking alone kills over 400,000 people each year. That's more people than AIDS, automobile accidents, homicides, suicides, drug overdoses and fires *combined!* A single puff of smoke contains carbon monoxide, benzene, formaldehyde (used to preserve dead animals and tissues in the lab), methanol (wood alcohol), acetylene (the fuel used in torches), ammonia, tar, nicotine and over 4,000 other chemicals, many of which are known to cause cancer.

This chemical cocktail doesn't just make you sick, it also makes you look old, ugly and smell bad. Through a variety of channels, smoking breaks down the collagen under your skin which causes increased wrinkling, it turns your skin, teeth and nails yellow, and gives you smoker's breath. The smoke sticks to your hair, skin, clothing and surroundings which make the rest of you smell bad too.

The sense of smell in most smokers is so impaired by their habit that they aren't aware of how they, their belongings and environments smell, but others are.

As bad as smoking may make you look on the outside, it's nothing compared to what it's doing to you on the inside. If you could turn yourself inside out and see what was happening to your heart and lungs it's doubtful that if you smoke, you would continue to do so, and if you don't, that you would ever start. I had the opportunity to have a representative from a local hospital bring an actual lung that had been removed from a cancer patient into my classroom to show my college students. The patient had been a smoker and also suffered from emphysema—another smoking related illness. It's one thing to hear about what smoking does to your body or to see a picture of it, but the impact of seeing the actual lung and what smoking had done to it was profound. Over half of the students in that class who had been smokers quit immediately and most were still smoke free by the end of the term. I wish every smoker or potential smoker could have the opportunity to see up close and realistically what smoking does to the body. If they could, there would probably be a lot less smokers.

PIPES AND CIGARS

Some people believe that pipe or cigar smoking is less harmful than cigarette smoking because not as much smoke is inhaled, but this is not correct, especially for someone who has previously been a cigarette smoker. Whether you are inhaling the smoke directly (which most previous cigarette smokers do), or indirectly from the air around you, you are still being affected by it. Inhaling second hand smoke which is a mixture of exhaled smoke from the tobacco user, and sidestream smoke emitted from the smoldering tobacco between puffs, is the third leading cause of lung cancer and it affects both adults and children who are exposed to it. The U.S. Surgeon General concluded that second-hand smoke causes lung cancer in adult non-smokers, and that children of parents who smoke have an increased frequency of respiratory symptoms and acute lower respiratory tract infections, as well as evidence of reduced lung function. It also aggravates allergies and asthma.

CHEWING TOBACCO

Chewing tobacco may be the worst of all. Smokeless tobacco, also known as snuff and chew, has the same negative effects on the body as smoking does, plus it greatly increases your risk of developing oral cancers, other diseases of the gums and mouth, and tooth loss. Most disturbing is the fact that a third of the 12 million Americans who use smokeless tobacco are under the age of 21.

All tobacco products contain nicotine and nicotine is a highly addictive substance. Once you begin using any type of tobacco it becomes difficult to stop. It's much easier to just not start in the first place.

HOW SMOKING AFFECTS YOUR HEALTH

Your Heart

Smoking damages the lining of your arteries, especially those that supply blood to your heart. This damage leads to the build up of plaque and narrowing of the arteries which increases your risk of having a heart attack. It also increases your heart rate, makes your blood platelets stickier and more likely to clot, raises your LDL, the bad cholesterol, and lowers your HDL, the good cholesterol.

Your Lungs

Your lungs are lined with tiny hair-like projections called cilia which sweep foreign particles and mucus towards the throat. The tar which cigarette smoke contains is a sticky resin like material that gums up the cilia impairing their ability to function and reducing the exchange of oxygen and carbon monoxide that normally takes place in your lungs. The resulting build up leads to the typical "smoker's cough," as well as increasing your risk for colds, bronchitis, and other respiratory infections. Exposure to the harmful chemicals in smoke causes lung cancer, cancer of the mouth, throat and esophagus. Eighty-five percent of all lung cancer is caused by smoking.

Other Cancers

You might expect that smoking would cause cancer in tissues that come in direct contact with the smoke like your throat or lungs, but smoking also increases your risk for cancer of the stomach, pancreas, bladder, kidney and cervix. It increases your risk for leukemia, rectal and colon cancer, and triples your risk for skin cancer.

Your Sex Life and Reproductive Problems

Smoking contributes to male impotence by reducing the blood flow to the penis and lowers sperm count and efficiency. It increases a woman's risk for ectopic pregnancy and miscarriage. Infants born to smoking mothers are at greater risk for stillbirth, prematurity, and low birth weight. Smoking also reduces folate levels, a B vitamin that reduces the risk of certain birth defects.

Your Bones

Smoking increases your risk for osteoporosis and hip fractures, and smokers are more likely to develop degenerative disorders of the spine.

Aging

Besides the effects on your skin, smokers have an increased risk for developing macular degeneration, cataracts, baldness and premature gray hair. It may also increase your risk of hearing loss and incontinence.

THE GOOD NEWS

Many of the effects of smoking can be reversed if you quit, regardless of your age. The sooner you stop, the sooner your body can start to recover.

20

MARIJUANA AND ALCOHOL

MARIJUANA: IT'S NOT THE 70'S ANYMORE

The primary mind-altering ingredient in marijuana (also known as grass, pot and weed) is THC, and depending on the type of plant, growing conditions, and the time of harvest, today's marijuana may contain as much as ten times more THC than did the marijuana available in the 1970's. This increase in potency increases the health risks of smoking marijuana, especially to the brain. Marijuana use changes the way the brain receives and acts on information. Regular use impairs concentration, learning, memory, and the ability to think clearly and solve problems.

The slowed thinking and reflexes caused by smoking marijuana severely impair a user's ability to drive a car safely. Research shows that a wide range of skills needed to drive are impaired for at least 4-6 hours after smoking a single marijuana cigarette, long after the "high" is gone. It can also lead to more aggressive behavior, especially in teens. THC is absorbed by most tissues and organs in the body, but it is mainly found in fat tissue. Urine tests can detect the metabolites of THC for up to a week after people have smoked marijuana. The "high" only lasts a short time, but the toxic chemicals remain in your body much longer.

The amount of tar inhaled by marijuana smokers and the level of carbon monoxide absorbed are three to five times *greater* than with tobacco. Marijuana smoke has also been found to contain more cancer causing agents than are found in tobacco. Someone who smokes marijuana regularly can develop the same respiratory problems as someone who smokes tobacco including coughing, emphysema and a greater frequency of respiratory infections such as colds. It can also increase your heart rate as much as 50 %.

People who smoke marijuana often experience episodes of extreme hunger called "the munchies" that can result is overeating and cause you to gain weight. It also impairs your judgment with regards to engaging in other risky behaviors, especially unprotected sex, and is considered a "gateway" drug that leads to the use of other, more dangerous drugs such as heroine, LSD, crack and cocaine.

If you want to give your brain a break, try exercising instead of smoking marijuana. It raises the level of endorphins and can produce a "natural high." Eating chocolate is a healthier substitute too. Chocolate contains chemicals similar to marijuana but without the negative side effects and it's also good for your heart. While the mind altering affects of exercise and eating chocolate aren't as strong as those associated with smoking marijuana, they are a whole lot better for your body and your health.

ALCOHOL: WHEN A BEVERAGE BECOMES A DRUG

Unlike tobacco and marijuana, alcohol has health benefits when consumed in moderation and it is usually considered part of the diet. That is why I included most of the information related to alcohol in the EAT section, but when alcohol is consumed in larger amounts, it is equally as dangerous to your health as any other drug, which is why it is included again here.

Moderation means up to two drinks per day for men and up to one drink per day for women and older adults. The recommendation is lower for women because they absorb alcohol more quickly than men, and their bodies' have a lower percentage of water than do men's, so alcohol remains more concentrated in women's bodies. Older adults tend to be more sensitive to the effects of alcohol and they often take more medications that can interact negatively with alcohol. Even over-the-counter drugs when combined with alcohol can be dangerous.

In greater concentrations, alcohol affects the brain similarly to marijuana, impairing thinking, judgment, coordination, and slowing reaction time, which is why it's the number one cause of traffic related fatalities. **Never drink and drive!** Consuming too much alcohol is bad for your health, but getting behind the wheel when you are intoxicated can be deadly for both you and others.

The effects of drinking while operating a boat are even more dramatic than when driving a car. According to the Office of Boating Safety, one-third the amount of alcohol that makes a person legally impaired on the road can make the same person equally impaired on the water due to a phenomenon called "boaters' hypnosis"—a kind of fatigue caused by motion, the effects of sun, heat, wind, glare and other aspects of the marine environment. And it doesn't just affect the driver. Passengers who have been drinking are more likely to fall overboard, even if the boat is not moving, and become disoriented and drown.

Like most drugs and toxins, alcohol puts extra strain on your liver. It increases the work load of this important organ while damaging it at the same time. Chronic excessive alcohol consumption can lead to cirrhosis and liver failure. Also like most drugs, alcohol can be addictive. Alcohol abuse and alcoholism destroys families, friendship, careers and lives. It's OK to drink in moderation, but if you can't drink moderately, don't drink at all.

21

OVER THE COUNTER MEDICATIONS

Just because you can buy them without a prescription doesn't mean that over-the-counter (OTC) medications are without risk. OTCs are generally considered safe when used according to instructions on the product label, but many people don't read those instructions and aren't aware of proper dosages, possible side effects, or potential interactions with other medications, drugs and foods. For example acetaminophen, a common pain reliever found in products such as Tylenol, can cause serious liver damage when taken in large quantities or by someone who also consumes alcohol regularly. The label clearly warns that "If you consume 3 or more alcoholic drinks every day, ask your doctor whether you should take acetaminophen or other pain relievers/fever reducers. Acetaminophen may cause liver damage" but many people don't take the time to read cautions such as these because they make the mistaken assumption that OTC's are always safe. Ibuprofen, another common pain reliever may cause drowsiness, dizziness, or blurred vision. Alcohol may intensify these effects increasing the risk of accidental injury. Use of alcohol during ibuprofen therapy increases the risk of stomach irritation and bleeding.

Before you use any medication, prescription or over-the-counter, *always* read the label carefully. Important information to look for includes:

- **Ingredients:** Check to make sure that you are using what you think you are, and that the product doesn't contain any ingredients that you are allergic to.
- **Dosage:** How much and how often should you take the product? Read the instructions carefully; the stronger or more concentrated the product is, the smaller the dose that is usually recommended. Always use appropriate measuring devices. A home utensil is not an accurate measure of a teaspoon or tablespoon.
- **Indications:** What is the product supposed to be used for?
- **Warnings:** Be aware of when you should stop taking the product, possible side effects, and when to see a health care provider.
- **Expiration date:** Medications should be properly disposed of after the expiration date.

Always examine product packaging carefully to make sure that it hasn't been tampered with. Don't buy a product if the package is damaged in any way. Always store medications in their original containers and don't take them in the dark. You may inadvertently grab the wrong container. Whether you take OTC's or prescription medications, always check with your health care provider or pharmacist regarding possible drug interactions.

Dispose of Outdated or
Unused Medications Properly!

Do not flush out-of-date or unused medication down the toilet, pour it down the sink, or put in the garbage. The active ingredients may contaminate ground water or lead to an increase in drug resistant microorganisms in the environment. Check to see if your pharmacy has a program that disposes of unused drugs in an environmentally safe manner. If your area does not have such a program, take the drugs to your municipality's waste disposal depot for proper disposal.

22

DIETARY SUPPLEMENTS AND HERBS

By definition a dietary supplement is a product intended to supplement the diet that contains one or more dietary ingredients. However, in practice many products are labeled as dietary supplements that aren't really dietary at all. They are more pharmaceutical in nature and function, but are marketed as dietary supplements because the legal restrictions and testing requirements aren't as stringent as those required for pharmaceuticals. Hormones such as DHEA and melatonin are such products. Herbs in their natural state or herbal supplements are often valued for their medicinal properties but may also be sold as dietary supplements.

"NATURAL" DOESN'T NECESSARILY MEAN "SAFE"

Many herbal products and dietary supplements are safe when used correctly and prudently, and I am a strong believer in their value in achieving optimum health and treating illness, but education with regard to their use is critical to ensure your safety.

Just because something is "natural" doesn't mean that it is safe. Mother Nature creates many substances that can be hazardous to human health (heroin for example). When using herbal products and dietary supplements, the burden of protecting yourself rests squarely on your own shoulders because these products are not regulated in the same way as conventional foods like fruits, vegetables, meats and grains, or pharmaceutical products are. Under the Dietary Supplement Health and Education Act of 1994 (DSHEA), the manufacturer of the product rather than a government agency is responsible for ensuring that it is safe. The FDA can only act after an unsafe product is in the marketplace. It is also up to the manufacturer to make sure that the information on the product label is truthful and not misleading.

In order to use these products safely, you must educate yourself and become a savvy consumer. For example, St. John's Wort is a popular herbal remedy for treating mild depression, but it can also increase your photosensitivity, making you more susceptible to skin damage from the sun. Ephedra, a common ingredient in weight loss and energy products can cause heart palpitations and has been associated with several deaths from heart attack and stroke. Comfrey, a plant traditionally used to treat external wounds, can damage your liver when taken internally, and fish liver oil may be contaminated with PCB's and other toxic chemicals.

Just as important as being aware of the risks of supplements is taking the time to fully understand them and how they should be used. The roots of the Kava plant have been used safely for centuries by the indigenous people of the islands of the South Pacific. Appreciated for its calming and soothing effects, Kava has been traditionally used as part of rituals and ceremonies after careful preparation. It was introduced into the US and European markets as a relaxant and a way to treat anxiety, but both the traditional form and usage were relatively ignored. Most of the kava available in stores is in capsules, and in order to keep prices down and meet demand, manufacturers have used the leaves and stems of the plant instead of just the roots. Unfortunately, the leaves and stems contain different chemicals and properties than do the roots, and usage of these plant components may lead to liver damage. Much of the calming affect of Kava in the traditional setting may also be related to the social support and interaction that occurs at gatherings, celebrations and rituals, something that is totally missing when you simply pop a pill. All dietary supplements have a correct and an incorrect way to be used.

Standardization of many herbal products is difficult, especially when they are still in their natural form because they are affected by variations in growing conditions and plant varieties. Just like a navel orange grown in one location may contain more Vitamin C than a valencia orange grown elsewhere, one type of chamomile may be much more potent than another type grown in a different location. It is limitations like this that make the use of natural products a little trickier than using carefully formulated and concentrated products that come with a complete instruction label.

The most important thing you can do to use dietary supplements successfully is to educate yourself. Before you begin taking any herb or dietary supplement, learn about what you are taking, how much to take, in what form, any possible side effects, and any possible interactions with other foods, drugs, or supplements. Also be sure to let your health care professional know what you are taking, especially if you have a medical condition, are taking medications, or are planning to have surgery.

23

PROTECTING YOUR BODY OUTDOORS

W hether you are working or playing outdoors it's important to be prepared for extreme weather conditions and to protect yourself from natural hazards. Each year many people are injured by exposure to cold temperatures, and heat related deaths are common in the summer months. Ticks and mosquitoes carry Lyme disease and the West Nile Virus, and excessive exposure to the sun can damage your eyes and cause skin cancer. When you are going to be outside, taking the right precautions can mean the difference between a pleasant walk in the park and a visit to the emergency room.

WATCHING OUT FOR WEATHER

When It's Cold Outside

In winter the two primary concerns are frostbite and hypothermia. Frostbite can occur quickly in extremely low temperatures or high wind conditions. If you feel any numbness or your skin begins to discolor and turn white, you need to get in from the cold as quickly as possible. Tobacco use can increase your risk of developing frost bite because it is a vasoconstrictor which causes your blood vessels to contract, reducing blood flow to the skin.

Hypothermia is an extremely dangerous condition in which your core body temperature begins to fall. It can make you feel sleepy and cause difficulty thinking, resulting in the "umbles"—stumbles, mumbles and fumbles which reflect changes in your motor coordination and level of consciousness. Unchecked, hypothermia can lead to serious injury and death. The best way to prevent hypothermia is to dress properly for the weather conditions, remain well fueled and fully hydrated, avoid getting wet, and don't use caffeine or alcohol. Caffeine is a diuretic which causes you to lose water making dehydration more likely. Alcohol is a vasodilator which causes your blood vessels to relax and open wider, increasing heat loss from your body. Even though alcohol may create a burning sensation and the illusion of warmth, consuming it when you are going to be exposed to cold temperatures is a dangerous thing to do. If you think that you are becoming hypothermic, seek shelter and assistance immediately.

Just like your car needs protection from the elements, so does your body. Layering loose fitting clothing works best. You can remove layers if you get warm and add them back on if the temperature begins to fall. The inner layer should be made of a fabric that draws perspiration away from your skin and the outer layer should be waterproof, wind resistant and breathable. When deciding on how many layers to wear, take wind conditions into consideration. If either you or the wind are moving fast, the result is the same, a substantial drop in how cold the air feels. This is the wind-chill factor. If the temperature is 32 degrees Fahrenheit and you are biking at 10 mph, the wind chill will make it feel like it is only 18 degrees. If you are biking on a breezy day against a 15 mph wind, the combined wind chill for 25 mph will make the temperature feel like it is below zero.

Mittens are warmer than gloves and don't forget your hat. You lose a great deal of heat through your head. Keeping your head covered can even help to keep your feet warm. Make sure that shoes or boots are large enough to allow for some trapped air between your foot and the shoe, and to allow for an extra pair of socks if it is needed.

Severe cold and bright reflected light can be damaging to your eyes. Wear goggles to prevent freezing of your corneas or sunglasses to prevent snow blindness.

When It's Hot Outside

Just as exposure to cold can cause injury and impair function, so can exposure to heat. Heat related illnesses include heat exhaustion, heat cramps and heat stroke. These illnesses can be extremely dangerous or even deadly. In the summer of 2003 a heat wave that struck France resulted in thousands of deaths caused by the elevated temperatures, especially among the elderly.

Heat exhaustion is a fluid depleted state with elevated body temperature that is characterized by fatigue, weakness, anxiety, confusion, headache, low blood pressure, dizziness, profuse sweating, and cold clammy skin. Heat exhaustion can be treated by cooling the body, lying flat with the head lower than the rest of the body and sipping cold beverages which contain electrolytes including sodium, potassium and magnesium. A sports drink is an example.

Heat cramps are severe muscle spasms caused by the loss of fluids and electrolytes. They often begin suddenly and affect hands, calves or feet. Heat cramps can be very painful and dis-abling as the muscles become hard, tense and difficult to relax. Heat cramps can be treated by consuming a cool, electrolyte containing beverage.

Heat stroke is a life threatening condition in which a person cannot sweat enough to cool the body. This condition can develop rapidly and requires immediate medical treatment. Symptoms of heat stroke include headache, vertigo, fatigue, disorientation and confusion, stumbling, clumsiness, loss of consciousness, and convulsions. The skin becomes hot, flushed, and dry, and both the heart rate and breathing rate increase.

All heat related illnesses begin with dehydration, so in order to prevent them be sure to consume enough fluids. If you are going to be exposed to extreme heat for long periods of time or you will be exercising in the heat, it's important to pre-hydrate before hand. Start drinking water two to three hours ahead of time to make sure that you are fully hydrated, and continue drinking at least every fifteen minutes during exposure or activity. Avoid strenuous activity in hot or humid weather if you can. If you can't, be sure to wear light colored clothing and a broad brimmed hat to protect your skin and reflect heat. You should always try to give your body time to adapt to the heat before beginning activity. Pay attention to your body and remain aware of how you are feeling at all times.

Avoiding Damage from the Sun's Rays

The warmth of the sun on your skin may feel wonderful and it can help your body to make Vitamin D, an essential nutrient, but basking in the sunshine for extended periods of time is not a good idea. Exposure to the ultraviolet rays of the sun ages your skin making it more wrinkled, and gives it a leathery texture. It also causes cancer and cataracts. Your best protection is to avoid excess exposure, but if you are going to be out in the sun, you can minimize the damage by wearing light colored protective clothing including a hat and sunglasses. To properly protect you eyes, be sure that your sunglasses block 99 percent of both UVA and UVB light.

If you are going to expose your skin to sunlight, your best defense against damage to is to wear a sunscreen with an SPF (sun protection factor) of 15 or more that blocks both UVA and UVB light. Frequent mistakes made by sun bathers are applying sunscreen too sparingly, and thinking that once they have applied sunscreen they are protected for the day. Sunscreen should be applied generously to dry skin 30 minutes before sun exposure and reapplied often, especially after swimming or excessive sweating. Waterproof and water-resistant sunscreens are best because their effectiveness is not reduced by perspiration.

Be aware that some medications can intensify the effects of the sun by causing photosensitivity. They can make your skin more sensitive to sunlight, increasing your risk of rashes, sunburn, blood vessel damage and cancer. Both prescription drugs and over the counter medications such as ibuprofen and antihistamines may cause this effect.

What Is SPF?

SPF stands for Sun Protection Factor and it tells you how much longer you can stay in the sun before burning than when you are not wearing a sunscreen. "SPF 15" means that you can stay in the sun 15 times longer than you could without sunscreen.

Hotter Than the Sun and Gone in a Flash—Lightning

According to The National Oceanic and Atmospheric Association, lightning strikes kill an average of 73 Americans each year and injure 300 others. It's the second leading weather-killer in the United States. While many lightning casualties happen as a storm is approaching, fifty percent of lightning deaths occur after the thunderstorm passes. Lightning can strike from long distances, so if storms are anywhere in the area it is important to take cover, even if the sky above you is clear. If you can see lightning, hear thunder, or the delay between the flash and the sound is less than 30 seconds, you are at risk.

Lightning Facts:

- One ground lightning strike can generate 100 million to 1 billion volts of electricity.
- The air within a lightning strike can reach 50,000 degrees Fahrenheit, which is hotter than the surface of the sun.
- The United States experiences over 25 million cloud-to-ground lightning strikes each year.

There is no place that is completely safe from lightning, but some places are safer than others. Inside of a sturdy building is the safest place to be during a storm, but don't use the telephone or be in contact with water or metal. Standing under a metal spigot taking a shower is not a good idea! Neither is sitting directly beneath a light fixture. If you are outdoors, an enclosed metal vehicle like a car or truck with the windows rolled up is your safest bet. Golf carts do not provide protection. Avoid being in or near high places, open fields, under trees, or anything metal such as light poles, bleachers or fences.

SMALL BUT DANGEROUS: TICKS AND MOSQUITOES

Most tick bites do not cause serious health problems, but some can. Ticks come in a variety of sizes and species, but most are very small; some like the deer tick which carries Lyme disease can be as small as the head of a pin. These spider-like insects fasten themselves onto skin and feed on blood. Normally they live in the fur and feathers of birds and animals, but they find humans pretty tasty too. The best way to prevent tick bites is to avoid wooded and grassy areas. If you are going to be in areas that are likely to contain many ticks, wear long pants and long-sleeved shirts that fit tightly at the ankles and wrists. Tuck your pants into your socks and wear closed shoes and a wide brimmed hat to protect your head. Ticks can be more easily spotted on light colored clothing than dark. Using an insect repellent that contains DEET can help prevent ticks from attaching to skin and clothing. Be sure to inspect your body carefully and have someone else check places like the back of your head that you can't see yourself.

If you find a tick it must be removed correctly. A tick will bury its head under your skin in order to "drink" blood. To minimize your risk of infection or disease, it is very important that you remove the tick alive and intact. If the tick is injured or killed it may regurgitate blood and disease causing organisms back into the wound. A detached head that remains in the skin can lead to infection.

Ticks can transmit several diseases including Lyme disease. Lyme disease often begins with a large red rash that looks like a "bull's eye" at the site of the bite, followed by flu-like symptoms and fatigue. Symptoms can occur anywhere from three to thirty days following infection. Lyme disease has been reported in almost every part of the country. If you think you may have been infected talk to your health care professional.

How To Remove A Tick

- Sterilize tweezers with alcohol or by exposing them to an open flame. Be sure the tweezers are cool before using them to remove the tick.
- Grasp the tick as close to its head as possible and pull back gently. In order to prevent the tick's body from separating from its head, do not rotate, twist, squeeze or pull too hard on the tick. You want the tick to let go on its own. Be patient.
- Once the tick lets go, make sure that it is intact and the head is still attached. If not, remove it.
- Disinfect the area.
- Save the tick in a plastic bag and mark the date on your calendar. Symptoms of Lyme disease may not appear for up to thirty days.

NOTE: Do not burn the tick with a hot match. This may cause the tick to regurgitate its contents back into your system, increasing your risk of disease.

In 1999 the West Nile virus arrived in the United States. Its primary means of transmission is through insects, particularly mosquitoes, so protecting yourself from bites has become of greater importance. The West Nile virus usually produces only mild symptoms including fever, headache and body ache, but it can also produce a more severe infection which can cause encephalitis. Encephalitis is inflammation of the brain and it can be fatal.

The best way to protect yourself against mosquito bites is to avoid being outdoors when mosquitoes are most active—at dawn, dusk and during a full moon. Wear light colored long pants and long-sleeved shirts when you are outside and spray both your clothing and skin with an insect repellent containing DEET. Avoid wearing floral scents and stay away from standing water.

Insect Repellent and Sunscreens

Insect repellent containing DEET can reduce the effectiveness of sunscreens. If you are going to be outdoors during the day and need both kinds of protection, choose a combination product. They are specially formulated for maximum protection from both insects and ultra violet rays.

24

AVOIDING EXPOSURE TO CHEMICALS

If you took the time to make a list of all of the chemical ingredients in every product that your body comes in contact with throughout the day, then added in the chemicals that you are exposed to via the air you breathe, the water you drink and the food you eat, you would probably be astounded at how much chemical exposure your body is subjected to daily. Most people think that the chemicals they use in everyday products have been adequately tested before being put on the market. The reality is that most are not. Many of the chemicals in commerce today lack basic testing data on potential health and environmental impacts. Some of these chemicals are known to be harmful and can have immediate and serious consequences for your health, others may not. Chemicals that you are exposed to everyday may fall into one of the following categories.

- Carcinogenic (cancer causing)
- Mutagenic (causes mutations in cells)
- Reproductive Toxin (linked to birth defects)
- Persistent (not easily excreted from the body)
- Bioaccumulative (magnifies up the food chain)
- Teratogenic (linked to birth defects)
- Endocrine Disruptor (disrupts the hormonal system)

Even when some of these chemicals are found in very small amounts which may pose no threat alone, no one is certain how the combined impact of all them may affect your health over time. It would be impossible to avoid all harmful chemicals entirely but there are steps you can take to reduce your exposure.

AIRBORNE TOXINS

Toxins arrive in the air from various sources both outside and inside of your home. Carbon monoxide results from the incomplete combustion of fuels. Outside, much of the carbon monoxide comes from automobile exhaust, but it is even more of a concern inside your home where it may come from appliances such as gas ranges, heaters, clothes dryers and fireplaces. About 200 deaths occur each year as a result of carbon monoxide poisoning.

Your furniture, carpeting and cabinetry can also give off harmful chemicals such as formaldehyde. Many aerosols, paints, solvents, and common household cleaning products contain hazardous ingredients and carry warning labels stating that they should be used only with adequate ventilation. Yet many homes lack adequate ventilation, especially those that are sealed as tightly as possible to prevent air leaks and keep energy costs down. Radon, a naturally occurring colorless, odorless, and tasteless radioactive gas can seep into your home from the earth below, and the harmful chemicals from tobacco products can build up as well. To reduce your exposure to airborne toxins in your home:

- Have all appliances and fireplaces checked by a qualified service person to make sure that they are in good working order and properly ventilated to the outside. Check frequently to make sure that the vents have not become blocked.

- Never start a vehicle or allow it to run in an enclosed space such as your garage with the door closed. Carbon monoxide levels build up quickly and can seep into your home.
- Never use a gas range or a gas oven to heat your home, even in a power outage. Avoid using kerosene or gas space heaters.
- Do not burn charcoal inside your home in a grill or in the fireplace.
- Have working carbon monoxide detectors and working smoke detectors in your home and don't forget to change their batteries at least once a year.
- Substitute common household ingredients such as salt, baking soda, white vinegar and borax in place of more toxic products. See table for suggestions.
- Read all labels and follow all directions on household cleaners and chemicals such as painting supplies, automotive supplies, and lawn and garden supplies. Use products only as intended and according to label instructions.
- Do not mix chemicals or cleaners. (Chlorine bleach when combined with ammonia creates fumes which can burn your lungs.)
- Wear gloves to avoid skin irritation or absorbing chemicals through your skin.
- Open a window, door, or vent whenever you are using chemical agents of any kind.
- Do not use products that require ventilation if no ventilation is available.
- Open your home regularly to "air it out," and help prevent the build up of toxins.

- Have your home tested for radon. Home test kits are available.
- Don't smoke or allow others to smoke in your home.
- Change air filters often.

Most air filters and purifiers are designed to remove particles, not gases. They can help to reduce the amount of smoke and dust in your air, but will not protect you from carbon monoxide, fumes or radon. Some plants like the spider plant can help to clean the air of toxic gases, but it takes a lot of plants to make a significant difference.

ENVIRONMENTALLY-SAFE INGREDIENTS

The common household ingredients below can be used as an alternative to commercial cleaners. Either combined, or on their own, they will produce safe and effective cleaners.

Baking Soda (sodium bicarbonate): An all-purpose, non-toxic cleaner, baking soda cleans, deodorizes, scours, polishes, and removes stains. Try leaving an open box in your refrigerator and in various locations around your home to absorb odors. Sprinkle on your carpets and then vacuum to deodorize them. Sprinkle in the bottom of trash cans and pour into drains and garbage disposals to reduce odors. Mix with water to form a paste and use for polishing silver and stainless steel.

Borax (sodium borate): Borax is a naturally occurring mineral made of sodium, boron, oxygen and water, and can usually be found in the laundry aisle of most grocery stores. It deodorizes, disinfects, removes stains and boosts the cleaning power of soap. It also prevents mold and odors and can kill ants, cockroaches, silverfish, and termites, but is non-toxic to humans. Use ¼ cup borax to ½ cup hot water as a disinfectant, add to your normal wash cycle to enhance cleaning, make a paste and use it in place of tub and tile cleaners, or sprinkle in areas where bugs and pests are a problem.

Lemon Juice: Cuts through grease and stains on aluminum and porcelain. Make a paste using salt to clean copper, or with 2 to 3 parts vegetable oil to make a polish for furniture and wood floors.

Pure Soap: Cleans everything.

Table Salt (sodium chloride): A mild disinfectant that can be used to make an abrasive, but gentle, scouring powder. Mix with equal parts flour and vinegar to clean brass.

Vinegar (dilute acetic acid): Removes mildew, stains, grease and wax buildup. Vinegar is a great glass cleaner; simply mix 5 tablespoons with 1 quart warm water. You can store it in a spray bottle for convenience. Vinegar can also be used to polish chrome.

Washing Soda (sodium carbonate): Cuts grease and disinfects. It will also increase the cleaning power of soap.

An all-purpose abrasive cleaner: Clean any surface with a mixture of baking soda and water or equal parts vinegar and salt. Be sure to rinse well. To make a milder abrasive, mix two parts borax with 1 part baking soda. You can store this mixture in a container with holes punched in the top to create a shaker for easy use.

Drain cleaner: To prevent clogs, once a week pour ¼ cup salt, ½ cup baking soda, and ½ cup vinegar down the drain. Allow it to stand for several minutes, then pour boiling water down the drain.

25

Food Safety

Toxins find their way into your body not only through the air you breathe but also through the water you drink and the foods you consume. Scientists believe that many synthetic chemicals can act as hormone disruptors—agents which can fool the body by imitating our natural hormones causing a wide array of health problems. To reduce your exposure to these products do the following:

- Drink filtered or purified water.
- Buy organic products whenever you can.
- Wash all fruits and vegetables thoroughly and peel any produce that has been waxed or oiled.
- Trim tops and outside leaves of leafy vegetables.
- Microwave food in ceramic or glass containers instead of plastic and never reuse the microwave plates that come with packaged or frozen foods. They are designed for one use only and can leach harmful products into your food when reused.
- Do not allow plastic wrap to come in contact with food when heated.
- Never allow non-stick pans to heat above 500° F or avoid

using them altogether. Use cookware with stainless steel surfaces and some healthy oils instead.

- Choose chlorine-free and unbleached paper products.

PREVENTING FOOD BORNE ILLNESS

More than 30 million Americans suffer from some type of food borne illness each year. While some people experience a day or two of gastrointestinal discomfort or temporary flu like symptoms, people who become seriously ill may live with the effects of food borne illness for years. Food poisoning can also be deadly. How you handle your food each step of the way, from where and how you purchase it, to the serving of leftovers is critical to keeping your food safe.

SAFE SHOPPING

Food safety begins at the point of purchase. Buying food that is fresh and has been properly stored is very important; so is making sure that your foods do not cross contaminate each other.

- Shop for meat, poultry and seafood last. Place it in plastic bags to keep it from dripping on other foods in your basket.
- Make sure that refrigerated foods are cold to the touch and frozen foods are rock solid. Partially defrosted or refrozen foods can be dangerous.
- Bring an ice chest or cooler to transport cold foods safely in hot weather, especially if the trip from grocery store to freezer will be more than a few minutes.
- Check the "sell by" date and don't purchase products with an expired date.

- Check to make sure that packaging is intact and sealed properly. Don't buy canned goods that are dented, rusted, cracked or have bulging lids.

SAFE STORAGE

Keep cold foods cold and hot foods hot. Warm is a comfortable temperature for humans but also for the bacteria that can grow in your food and make you sick. Check your freezer with a thermometer to make sure that it is at or below 0° F and your refrigerator is below 40° F. Space items far enough apart to allow air to circulate freely. When holding warm food for serving make sure that it is above 140° F.

- Freeze fresh meat, poultry and seafood immediately if you don't plan to use it within a few days. Always wrap tightly or seal in air tight containers.
- Thaw frozen foods in the refrigerator and marinate foods there as well, not on the counter or in the sink.
- Meat, fish and poultry stored in the refrigerator should be wrapped tightly or in a waterproof container to prevent juices from dripping.
- Store meat, fish and poultry separately from fresh fruits and vegetables. Especially those that won't be cooked before serving.
- Use refrigerated meats and deli products within 3–4 days.
- Store eggs in their carton inside the refrigerator rather than on the door.

PREPARING TO COOK

Before you begin to cook, it's important to make sure that everything you are going to use in food preparation is clean and ready to go.

- Wash your hands thoroughly with hot soapy water before you begin handling food, between touching different types of food, and after you pause and engage in any other activity. Be especially careful after blowing your nose, using the bathroom, changing a diaper, or touching pets.
- Cover any wounds or sores on your hands or wear gloves to protect you and your food.
- Wash all surfaces and utensils that you will be using. Use clean cloths, towels and sponges. Microwave your dish sponge for one minute to kill bacteria that it may be harboring.
- Keep raw, cooked and ready to eat food separated. Never chop fruits and vegetables on a cutting board or with the same knife that has been used for meat products without washing and sanitizing thoroughly. A solution of 1 Tbsp. chlorine bleach to 1 gallon of water works well.
- Check all foods, especially meats, poultry and seafood for freshness. Spoiled food doesn't always smell bad or look bad, but if it does smell bad or look bad, it is bad. ***When in doubt, throw it out!***
- Wash all fruits and vegetables thoroughly under running water, even if you plan to peel or cut them. Otherwise the bacteria and contaminants on the outside can be transferred to the inside. Remove outer leaves and separate inner ones well when washing leafy vegetables.

Cook to the Correct Temperature

Use a digital or dial food thermometer to ensure that meats are completely cooked. Insert the thermometer into the center of the food and wait 30 seconds to ensure an accurate measurement.

- Beef, lamb, and veal should be cooked to at least 145° F; pork and ground beef to 160° F; whole poultry and thighs to 180° F; poultry breasts to 170° F; and ground chicken or turkey to 165° F.
- Seafood should be thoroughly cooked to an internal temperature of at least 145° F. Fish that's ground or flaked, such as a fish cake, should be cooked to at least 155° F and stuffed fish to at least 165° F
- Eggs should be cooked until the white and the yolk are firm. Avoid foods containing raw eggs, such as homemade ice cream, mayonnaise, eggnog, cookie dough and cake batter, they may be contaminated with Salmonella. Cooking the egg-containing product to an internal temperature of at least 160° F will kill the bacteria.
- Cook stuffing separately. If you do cook it inside of meat or poultry, stuff it loosely just before cooking and make sure the temperature reaches 165° F.
- Do not partially cook foods and then refrigerate or set aside until later. They may not reach a high enough temperature to kill bacteria.
- Don't contaminate cooked meat by placing it on a platter that was used for raw meat. Don't use marinade or sauces that have been in contact with raw foods without boiling them for at least one minute.
- Stir or rotate foods when microwaving to assure even heating.

SERVING

Keep foods in the safe temperature ranges until you are ready
to serve them. That means they should be hotter than 140° F or
colder than 40° F.

- Use clean utensils and serving dishes for cooked food.
  Never use the same unwashed utensils or serving dishes
  that were used for raw meats, poultry, or fish.
- Don't allow food to remain at room temperature for more
  than 2 hours.

HANDLING LEFTOVERS

Cover and refrigerate leftovers quickly and reheat thoroughly
before serving again. Leftovers should be tightly wrapped or
placed in sealed containers and stored in the refrigerator as
soon as possible. When you are ready to eat them, reheat to at
least 165° F before serving. Freeze leftovers that you won't be
using in the next few days.

For more information about food safety, contact: The U.S.
Food and Drug Administration Food Information Line at (888)
SAFE FOOD.

26

GENERAL SAFETY GUIDELINES

Following a few simple guidelines can go a long way towards keeping you healthy and safe. To prevent illness and stop the spread of infections, the most important thing you can do is wash your hands frequently. Wash them after you use the bathroom, cough, or sneeze. Wash them both before and after handling foods. Also wash them if you have been using cleaning agents or chemicals or have touched contaminated surfaces. Proper hand washing involves using soap, rubbing your hands together vigorously for several seconds and rinsing with lots of running water. A quick rinse is better than nothing, but it won't offer you much protection. The more often and thoroughly you wash your hands the better off you will be, and the less likely you are to spread germs to others.

Many accidents and injuries can be prevented by taking simple precautions and using common sense. To help protect yourself:

- Always wear a seat belt while in a car and be sure that children are properly restrained using a car or booster seat.
- Always wear a safety helmet when riding on a motorcycle, bicycle, skateboard or when rollerblading.

- Never drink or use drugs when you drive and never drive when you are overtired.
- Keep the temperature of your hot water heater lower than 120 degrees Fahrenheit to prevent burns, especially for children and the elderly.
- Always wear a life jacket when engaging in water activities such as boating or jet skiing.
- Secure all ladders and don't use them near electrical lines.
- Clean spills immediately to prevent slips and falls.
- Wear eye protection and earplugs when using power tools or lawn equipment.

PART THREE:

PREVENTATIVE MAINTENANCE

Every automobile manufacturer includes in their operating instructions a recommended schedule of maintenance for their vehicles. This maintenance schedule lets you know what you need to do and when, in order to keep your car running in peak condition, to prevent problems, and to help your vehicle last as long as possible. It includes information such as when to change the oil, how often to rotate the tires, and when to have the brakes, hoses and lines checked. The more mileage your car accrues, the more maintenance and inspections that are recommended. Properly maintaining your body also requires not only the daily care of eating a healthy diet, getting enough activity and exercise, relaxing, and getting enough sleep, but regular service and inspections as well. And just like your car, the older your body is, the more service and maintenance it too will require.

The maintenance schedule for your body is meant to ensure early detection of health problems and allow for preventative measures or the early treatment of disease. Early intervention is very important in determining the outcome of an illness. The earlier a problem is uncovered and treatment begun, the better your chances will be for a full recovery. Neglecting to take your car in for service can lead to unnecessary damage to your vehicle and costly repairs down the road. Neglecting to take your body in for recommended tests and screenings can also lead to unnecessary damage and costly repairs, but it also might cost you your life.

The guidelines included in this manual are intended for generally healthy adults. If you are not feeling well, suspect that you may have a health issue, have a current medical condition or are at an increased risk for developing one, you should see your health care provider for appropriate guidelines.

PREVENTATIVE MAINTENANCE SCHEDULE

Who Needs It	What You Need	How Often You Need It	Additional Information
All Adults	Blood Pressure Measurement	Every 2 years	
All Adults	Comprehensive Eye Exam	Every 2-3 years	Exam should include testing for glaucoma and frequency should increase to annually after age 65.
Women over 18	Clinical Breast Exam	Every 3 years	This should be done as part of a regular health exam by a health professional.
Women over 21	Pap smear	Every 1 - 3 years	This test should be performed sooner and more often if you are sexually active or have multiple partners. Talk with your health care professional.

Men 35 and over Women 45 and over	Cholesterol Measurement	Every 5 years	If you have a family history of heart disease, you have diabetes, or you smoke, talk with your health care professional.
Women 40 and over	Mammogram	Every year	
	Height Measurement	Every year	A loss in height may be a warning sign of osteoporosis.
Adults over 50	Colorectal Cancer Test	Occult blood test annually	A baseline sigmoidoscopy should be performed. It should be repeated as recommended by your health care professional.
Adults over 50 year	Flu vaccine	Every year	
Adults over 65	Pneumonia vaccine	At least once	
Women over 65	Bone density test	Every 2 years	

ADDITIONAL TESTING THAT MAY BE RECOMMENDED

If you have experienced signs of depression for more than two weeks such as feelings of sadness, hopelessness, or have lost interest in doing things, you should be screened by your health care professional for depression. If you have high cholesterol or high blood pressure, you should also be screened for diabetes.

WHAT ABOUT AN ANNUAL PHYSICAL EXAM?

Most of us are creatures of habit and there are many things that we do just because we have always done them, not necessarily because they are necessary to do or the right thing to do. Having an annual physical for healthy adults who have no symptoms of illness is one of those things. Many years of study and research have found no evidence to support that having an annual exam, or many of the tests normally included in one, is necessary or beneficial. As a result, the most recent guidelines from the U.S. Department of Health and Human Services Agency for Healthcare Research and Quality does not include annual physicals in its recommendations. Occasionally a health issue that isn't yet causing any symptoms may be discovered during a routine physical exam, but this doesn't take place frequently enough to justify the time, resources, or potential risks from unnecessary testing involved in annual physicals to recommend them for everyone. Having a physical is a great way to establish a relationship with a health care professional so that you have one when you need one, and if it makes you feel more comfortable and secure to visit your health care professional regularly, then having an annual physical may be worthwhile for you as an individual. If you are experiencing any health related problems or symptoms, don't wait for a routine exam, contact your healthcare professional right away.

WHAT ABOUT SELF EXAMS?

It is important to know your body so that you can more readily detect any signs, symptoms or changes that may develop. This applies to your whole body including, but not limited to, your skin, breasts and testicles. It is equally important however to understand the limitations of self examinations and not use them as a replacement for professional exams or screening tests. Many people do not perform self exams correctly, and even when they are performed correctly, they cannot detect problems as early as some clinical tests can. Knowing how your breasts or testicles normally look and feel is valuable as long as you don't allow a "normal" self exam to give you a false sense of security that prevents you from seeing your health care professional when you should.

28

TUNE UPS

S ome types of preventative care can be very helpful at preventing illness or just helping your body to run more efficiently. Acupuncture, chiropractic, and massage therapy are
medical disciplines that focus on wellness and improving the
overall function of the body as much as they do on repairing it
should it become damaged or ill. Massage therapy is discussed
in the RELAX section.

ACUPUNCTURE

Acupuncture is a form of energy medicine that has been
practiced for thousands of years in the Orient and is recognized
by the National Institutes of Health as an effective form of
medical treatment for a variety of conditions. Its primary goal is
to keep the body's energies flowing smoothly and to bring them
all into balance. An energy imbalance can manifest itself as
chronic pain, fatigue or general malaise. It can also lead to serious illness. Many things can create imbalances in the body's
energies such as an unhealthy lifestyle, environmental pollu-
tants, illness or trauma. Even if you feel fine and your body
seems to be running well, the day to day stresses of life may be
causing you to function at less than your peak performance

levels. An acupuncture treatment, like a tune up, can improve that performance and help you to feel even better.

CHIROPRACTIC

Chiropractic emphasizes the relationship between structure and function in the body. Doctors of chiropractic believe that good health depends, in part, on the normal alignment of the body's parts, and that misalignment can be a major factor in pain, illness and performance. When the wheels of your car become misaligned, you can still drive, but the wear and tear on your tires is increased, steering becomes more difficult, and your ride won't be as smooth. When parts of your body become misaligned, they don't move smoothly either and can cause undue stress on muscles, tendons, ligaments and other types of soft tissue. Proper alignment of the spine is considered of special importance because of its central role in the functioning of the nervous system, which in turn affects the health of every other system in the body. Many things can lead to misalignments in the structure of your body including exercise, injury, or even the way you walk and sit. A chiropractic adjustment to correct these misalignments can contribute greatly to your overall wellbeing.

29

Taking Care of Your Teeth

Good oral health care is important to your teeth and to your general health. With proper care, you teeth will last you for life. You should brush you teeth with a soft or medium bristled toothbrush at least twice a day or after meals, and floss daily. Don't smoke or chew tobacco and limit the amount of sweets you eat between meals. You should see your dentist or dental hygienist regularly for professional cleaning of your teeth. Even with regular brushing and flossing, plaque can build up and harm your teeth and your gums. Gum disease can increase your risk of heart disease, so taking care of your teeth helps take care of your heart too.

30

HEART HEALTH

Heart Disease is the leading cause of death in adults over 35 years of age. It affects about 58 million people, claims almost three quarters of a million lives each year, and represents over 200 billion dollars in costs annually. What's truly amazing is that much of this suffering and expense is preventable. Recent research has shown that approximately 90 percent of all people who develop heart disease have at least one of four risk factors. They smoke, have high blood pressure, elevated cholesterol levels, or suffer from diabetes—all of which can be eliminated or improved through lifestyle changes and medical treatment.

For years it was assumed that the greatest risk factors for heart disease were age, sex, and heredity. You developed heart disease because you were a male, a post-menopausal woman, getting older, or because it ran in your family—all things which you couldn't do anything about. If this were indeed the case, efforts to reduce your risk of heart disease would be limited in their ability to prevent illness. However, our current understanding of what leads to heart disease lends itself to a far more positive outlook. You can't control or affect your genetic makeup or how old you are, but you can make choices and seek treatments which can dramatically affect each of the "big four" risk factors, as well as the lesser but still important ones including homocysteine levels, stress, lack of exercise, and being overweight. Your family history and age are still important considerations, but the focus has shifted from things you can't control to things you can.

Heart disease encompasses a variety of different disorders of the cardiovascular system. The following explanations of a few of these conditions may be helpful in understanding why certain behaviors put you at increased risk for specific problems.

Atherosclerosis: Also called hardening of the arteries, atherosclerosis results primarily from your body's efforts to repair injuries and damage to your blood vessels. Your blood vessels, including your arteries, are the highways of your body's transportation system. Just like real highways, they can become damaged over time, especially by high blood pressure and other irritants which create the equivalent of pot holes. Your body repairs these "pot holes" in your cardiovascular highway by laying down fatty plaque. Just as repaired roads become bumpy, so do repaired vessels. Instead of a smooth surface for blood to flow over, the lining of the vessels develops rough spots which tend to collect debris. These bumps and debris build up over time causing the blood vessels to become narrower and more rigid, making it easier for them to become blocked by clumps of floating material or blood clots. When a blood vessel becomes blocked, all of the tissue that is on the far side of the obstruction is denied blood and oxygen and quickly dies. If this blockage occurs in one of the arteries delivering blood to your heart, you have a heart attack. If it occurs in one of the blood vessels in your brain, you have a stroke.

Coronary Artery Disease (CAD): CAD begins with atherosclerosis in the arteries which deliver blood and oxygen to the heart. Even though the heart is filled with blood, it cannot use that blood for its own nourishment. It must depend on the coronary arteries to meet its needs. As with any atherosclerosis, CAD develops gradually as fatty plaques become deposited on the lining of the vessels causing them to become narrower and restricting blood flow. Eventually the plaque calcifies, causing the arteries to become harder and stiffer. Left untreated, CAD can eventually lead to heart failure or a heart attack. These are sometimes preceded by chest pain (angina) and fatigue, but may also occur without warning.

Cardiac Arrhythmias: An arrhythmia is an irregular heartbeat caused by a problem with the heart's electrical system. It's similar to the timing being off in your car's engine. Arrhythmias can be caused by many things including caffeine, alcohol, smoking, stress or serious heart conditions. Many arrhythmias are brief and unnoticeable, but others can be startling, or even fatal.

THE RISK FACTORS FOR HEART DISEASE

There are ten significant risk factors for heart disease. Each is an independent risk factor on its own, but several also contribute to the development of other risk factors. For instance, obesity and smoking are both risk factors for heart disease, and both can increase your cholesterol levels and your blood pressure which are also risk factors for heart disease. This makes obesity and smoking especially dangerous, but it also means that when you address them by losing weight or stopping smoking, it can be doubly beneficial to your heart.

RISK FACTOR: SMOKING AND EXPOSURE TO SECOND HAND SMOKE

As you discovered in the Safety Precautions section, smoking and exposure to second hand smoke contribute to heart disease in a number of ways. They raise your level of bad cholesterol (LDL), lower your level of good cholesterol (HDL), encourage atherosclerosis, reduce oxygen availability, and increase your heart rate.

What You Can Do About Smoke

If you are a smoker, quit! There are many effective tools to assist you in this quest, from support groups to medications. If you don't smoke, do whatever you can to reduce your exposure to second hand smoke. Many states including California and Florida have taken steps to try and protect you by not allowing smoking in public places like restaurants. If your state doesn't regulate public smoking, avoid locations and establishments where smoking is permitted. Sitting in a non-smoking section is better than nothing, but it may provide little protection if it is located near a smoking section or shares a ventilation system with one.

RISK FACTOR: HIGH BLOOD PRESSURE (HYPERTENSION)

Narrowing of your blood vessels requires your heart to pump with more force in order to deliver blood throughout your body. Just like a garden hose, the narrower the opening through which your blood must move, the greater the pressure that will build up. Untreated, hypertension will cause the heart to eventually overwork itself to the point where serious damage can occur. The heart muscle can thicken and become less efficient, and increased pressure can injure the lining of blood vessels leading to increased atherosclerosis, which in turn increases your risk of having a heart attack or a stroke. Hypertension can also lead to injury of the brain, the eyes, and the kidneys.

Blood pressure is measured as the heart contracts (your

systolic pressure) and relaxes (your diastolic pressure). Blood pressure is considered normal if your systolic pressure is below 120 mm Hg and your diastolic pressure is below 80 mm Hg. Pre-hypertension is represented by a systolic pressure of 120 to 139 mm Hg or a diastolic pressure of 80 to 89 mm Hg. A reading of 140/90 to 159/100 is considered moderately high, 160/100 to 179/109 is considered very high, and 180/ 110 or above is dangerously high.

What You Can Do About High Blood Pressure

Following the guidelines for diet, exercise, stress management, and rest in the Basic Operating Instructions will go a long way in treating hypertension. A diet lower in salt and higher in potassium, magnesium, calcium, Vitamin C, Vitamin E and the B vitamins has been shown to reduce blood pressure. The recommendations in the EAT section will help you to achieve this. So will following the DASH (Dietary Approaches to Stop Hypertension) diet which is very similar. Regular exercise helps to regulate blood pressure also. With hypertension, the regularity of the exercise is more important than the intensity. The key is not how hard you exercise, but to do it consistently and frequently.

Eating right and exercising regularly will also help you to achieve and maintain a healthy weight. Being overweight increases your blood pressure and is also an independent risk factor for heart disease. Emotional factors play an important role in the development of hypertension too. Studies have shown that the regular use of stress management techniques like those described in the RELAX section have been associated with reducing blood pressure to healthy levels. But perhaps the most important lifestyle choice you can make is to not smoke. Nicotine is a vasoconstrictor. It causes your blood vessels to contract and narrow, further restricting blood flow and increasing blood pressure.

Many people who follow all of these instructions can lower their blood pressure significantly without further intervention. But high blood pressure is very dangerous, so it is important to discuss all of your options with your health care professional. There are effective medications which can lower your blood pressure including diuretics, alpha, beta, and calcium channel blockers, ACE inhibitors, and others.

RISK FACTOR: ELEVATED CHOLESTEROL LEVEL

Cholesterol is a waxy, fat-like substance that you consume by eating animal products such as meat, eggs and dairy food, but most of the cholesterol in your body, about 80%, is produced by your liver. Despite its reputation for being a contributor to heart disease, cholesterol is actually necessary to good health. Cholesterol is used in the making of Vitamin D and in the metabolism of carbohydrates and proteins. It is part of every cell wall and is used to make bile, a substance that helps you to digest fat. Because fats and water don't mix well, cholesterol must be "packaged" for transport through your blood stream to prevent it from clumping together the way oil does on top of soup. The body packages cholesterol in lipoproteins.

Low-density lipoproteins (LDL) contain lots of fat and break apart easily. They stick to the lining of your arteries causing damage and making the artery narrower. Areas of damage tend to attract other substances like blood cells and clotting materials that combine to form plaque and eventually harden the arteries. That is why LDL is considered the "bad cholesterol," (LDL is Lousy so the Lower your level, the better). VLDL or Very Low

Density Lipoproteins (*Very Lousy*) are even worse. Intermediate-density lipoproteins (IDLs) are a type of cholesterol that seems to raise the risk of non-fatal heart attacks and angina (chest pain), and Lipoprotein-a (Lp(a)) and Apolipoprotein B (apo-B) are other types of lipoproteins associated with an increased risk of heart disease. Chylomicrons are used to transport triglycerides, the form of fat that your body stores in fat tissue.

At the other end of the spectrum are High- Density lipoproteins (HDL). HDLs act like a cleaning service picking up the trash—in this case cholesterol—and transporting it back to the liver for disposal. They help to prevent heart disease rather than increasing your risk of developing it. HDL is often referred to as "good" cholesterol, therefore the *H*igher your *H*DL level is, the *H*appier you should be.

Keeping your total cholesterol level in check is very important but equally important may be your ratio of "good" HDL cholesterol to "bad" LDL cholesterol. Your cholesterol ratio is your total cholesterol number divided by your HDL cholesterol number; a ratio of less than 5:1 is preferred. The lower your ratio is, the lower your risk of developing heart disease. Total cholesterol levels of less than 200 mg/dL are considered desirable, levels between 200 to 239 mg/dL are borderline high, and levels above 240 mg/dL are high. Your LDL cholesterol should be less than 130 mg/dL and ideally your HDL should be greater than 45 mg/dL. Your triglyceride level should be less than 150 mg/dL.

What You Can Do About High Cholesterol

Your first line of defense against elevated cholesterol levels is making healthy lifestyle choices. You should avoid smoking and second hand smoke, trans fatty acids, saturated fats, and cholesterol in your diet. You need to make sure you get enough omega-3 fatty acids, eat enough fiber, get enough exercise, and maintain a healthy weight. An explanation of the different types of fat is covered in the EAT section, as are the benefits of dietary fiber.

Trans fatty acids are primarily found in partially hydrogenated oils and the products made from them. Saturated fats and cholesterol primarily come from animal products such as meat, poultry, eggs, and dairy products. You can help to reduce your cholesterol levels by replacing meats with vegetable sources of protein such as soy, beans and nuts. The National Cholesterol Education Program suggests limiting cholesterol intake to less than 200 mg per day.

To increase your intake of omega-3 fatty acids, eat fish at least 2-3 times per week, consume flaxseed or its oil regularly, or take a fish oil or flaxseed supplement. To get enough fiber, eat more fruits, vegetables, and whole grains. The soluble fiber found in foods like oatmeal binds with cholesterol in your gastrointestinal tract preventing its absorption into the body. Eating more fiber will make you feel full which can also help you to lose weight.

If lifestyle changes such as lowering your fat intake, increasing your exercise level, and losing weight do not sufficiently lower your cholesterol, cholesterol lowering drugs such as statins may be necessary. Talk to your health care professional to see whether or not they are appropriate for you.

Risk Factor: Diabetes

There are two types of diabetes; juvenile or type 1, and adult onset or type 2. Type 1 diabetes usually occurs before the age of thirty and is characterized by insufficient, or the complete absence of insulin, the hormone necessary for managing blood sugar. For unknown reasons that may be genetic or environmental, the immune system attacks the pancreas and destroys the beta cells which make insulin. Insulin must be taken regularly by injection in order for the body to be able to process carbohydrates and survive. This type of diabetes is also known as Insulin Dependent Diabetes Mellitus or IDDM.

In type 2 diabetes the pancreas is able to make insulin but the cells do not recognize or respond to it normally. It is most often associated with being overweight. Until recently this form of diabetes was uncommon before the age of thirty, but with the dramatic increase in obesity it is affecting younger and younger individuals, even teenagers.

What You Can Do About Diabetes

There is nothing that you can do to prevent type 1 diabetes, but it can be treated very successfully through a combination of insulin injections and diet. Type 2 diabetes is usually associated with excess body fat so the most important thing you can do is to lose weight. For some people losing sufficient weight can return insulin function and blood sugar levels to normal. If glucose levels remain high, medication may be necessary to bring them under control and prevent permanent damage to the body, especially the cardiovascular system, the eyes, and kidneys. Two out of three people with diabetes die from heart disease.

RISK FACTOR: ELEVATED HOMOCYSTEINE LEVEL

Homocysteine is an amino acid (a building block of protein) that is a natural byproduct of the breakdown of methionine, an essential amino acid found mainly in meat. There is increasing evidence that when homocysteine levels rise too high it can increase your risk of developing atherosclerosis by damaging the arteries and increasing levels of LDL. It may also increase your risk of having a heart attack.

What You Can Do About Homocysteine

Your body requires B vitamins to convert homocysteine back into methionine or into simpler amino acids that the body can easily dispose of. The three vitamins of concern are Vitamin B_6, Vitamin B_{12}, and folic acid (folate). Eating a diet high in fruits, vegetables and whole grains should supply sufficient quantities of these vitamins to prevent your homosysteine level from rising above normal. A multiple vitamin and mineral supplement that contains 400 mcg of folate can be taken as insurance, but large quantities of B vitamins are not necessary.

RISK FACTOR: C-REACTIVE PROTEIN (CRP)

CRP is made in the liver in response to inflammation somewhere in the body and is necessary for fighting injury and infection. It also rises in response to inflammation of blood vessels. Cholesterol causes plaque to build up in blood vessels, but heart attacks and strokes are usually triggered when inflammation causes a piece of plaque to break off and block an artery. CRP levels often rise many years before a first heart attack or stroke occurs and may be an indicator that you are at increased risk for coronary artery disease.

What You Can Do About CRP

The same strategies that reduce cholesterol appear to lower CRP levels. These include avoiding the use of tobacco products, losing weight, exercising, and the use of statin drugs.

RISK FACTOR: OBESITY

Being overweight increases your risk for developing hypertension, elevated cholesterol levels, and diabetes. Keeping your larger body supplied with blood also puts an extra burden on your heart. In addition to how much fat your body has stored, where that excess fat is located also seems to be important. People who store fat primarily on the upper or middle part of their bodies (central adiposity) seem to be at the greatest risk for developing heart disease and diabetes. These people are often referred to as "apples." Storing fat on the hips and thighs doesn't appear to raise the risk of heart disease as much. These people are referred to as "Pears."

What You Can Do About Obesity

Obesity is a complex issue with many contributing factors. It's easier to prevent weight gain than to lose weight so if you are not overweight now, work hard to stay that way. If you are overweight, following the guidelines in the Basic Operating Instructions section will help you to bring your weight under control and maintain a healthy weight. Fad diets and yoyo dieting are not healthy for your body or your heart. Some studies suggest that repeated weight loss may even be worse for you than remaining overweight. However a lifestyle that is focused on wellness naturally supports a healthy body weight. You don't have to focus on "losing" weight. If you set your sights on "gaining health" instead, attaining a healthy weight will be a natural byproduct of your healthier lifestyle. It is a positive approach that you can live with for the rest of your life.

RISK FACTOR: SEDENTARY LIFESTYLE

Your heart is a muscle and just like any other muscle, it needs exercise to remain fit. If you don't use it, you lose it. The walls of your arteries also contain muscle, and the action of skeletal muscles helps smaller veins like those in your legs to carry blood back to your heart. Without activity or exercise all of these muscles can become weaker and less efficient. A sedentary lifestyle also makes it much easier to gain weight and more difficult to lose it.

What You Can Do About a Sedentary Lifestyle

If you have been a long term couch potato, start out slowly by just getting moving. Go for regular walks or participate in activities that require you to stand and move rather than sit. As your body becomes more acclimated to moving, increase your activity level. While all activity is helpful, aerobic exercise is unique in its ability to improve cardiovascular fitness. If you are overweight or have problems with arthritis or pain, water aerobics can help bring your heart rate up without putting too much stress on your joints. For complete guidelines on getting your body moving, see the MOVE section of Basic Operating Instructions.

RISK FACTOR: STRESS

Too much stress causes your body to respond as if it's in an emergency situation. Your heart rate increases, your blood pressure increases and your blood platelets become stickier and more likely to clot. All of these events contribute to the development of heart disease, especially if they become a routine part of your daily life. If you tend to overeat when you are stressed, it can also lead to weight gain.

What You Can Do About Stress

Recognize that stress is an important health issue not just a state of mind, then take a deep breath, and follow the guidelines in the RELAX section. They will help you to reduce the amount of stress in your life and its impact on your health.

RISK FACTOR: OBSTRUCTIVE SLEEP APNEA (OSA)

Obstructive sleep apnea can lead to an increase in blood pressure. If the condition is severe enough it can also cause the left side of the heart to become enlarged. Obstructive sleep apnea occurs when soft tissue falls back and blocks the airway resulting in a stoppage of breathing. When the brain detects a drop in oxygen it triggers the body to gasp for air, resulting in the loud snoring or gasping sounds common to this disorder. The repeated struggle to breathe causes tension in the left ventricle and increases the heart rate. OSA has been found in as many as 50% of individuals with heart failure.

What You Can Do About OSA

See your health care professional. There are effective treatments, such as continuous positive airflow pressure machines which deliver air through a mask over your nose to help you breathe regularly while you are asleep. OSA is more common in obese individuals so if you are overweight, losing weight may be valuable.

DOES AN ASPIRIN A DAY KEEP A HEART ATTACK AWAY?

Regular use of low dose aspirin can significantly reduce the risk of coronary heart disease in some people, but it isn't without risks. Aspirin can increase gastrointestinal bleeding and

cause bleeding in the brain. It can also interact with other medications, both prescription and over-the-counter. Talk to your health care professional to determine if an aspirin a day is right for you.

TAKE CARE OF YOUR TEETH, IT'S GOOD FOR YOUR HEART

Researchers have found that people with periodontal disease are almost twice as likely to suffer from coronary artery disease as those without periodontal disease, so brush, floss and see your dentist for regular cleanings.

INDEX

For more information about
Speaking of Wellness seminars,
programs and books please visit our website
www.speakingofwellness.com

Speaking of Wellness
PMB #202
2200 Winter Springs Blvd. Suite 106
Oviedo, Florida 32765
USA
Tel: (407) 366-6337